THE PEOPLE

Date & Time:

Birth Number:

Location / Setting:

Mother:

Partner:

Baby:

Baby's Sex:

Maternal Age:

Gestation:

Length of Labor:

Baby's Weight & Apgars

Pregnancy Notes:

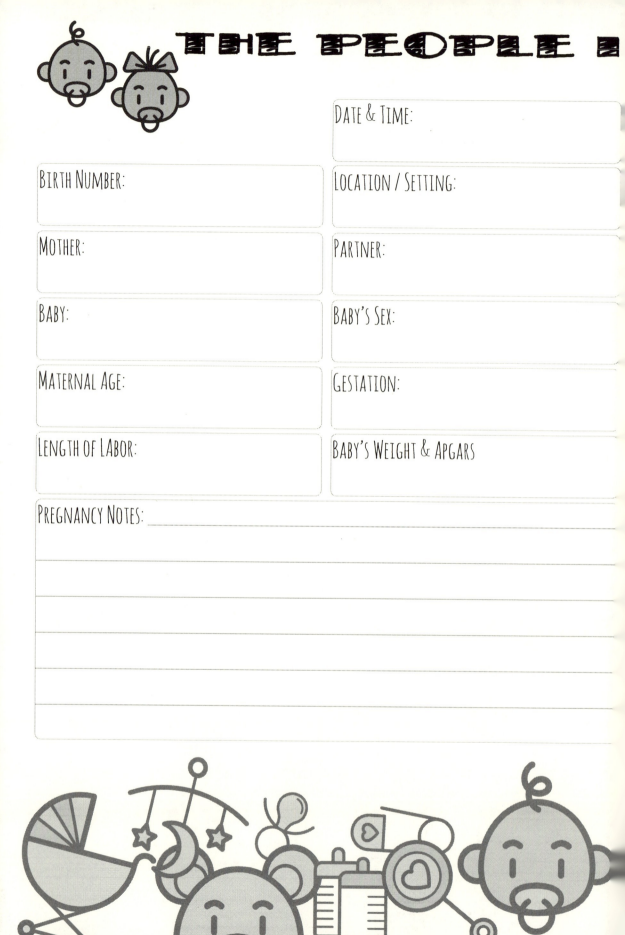

HAVE HELPED OUT

COMMENTS:

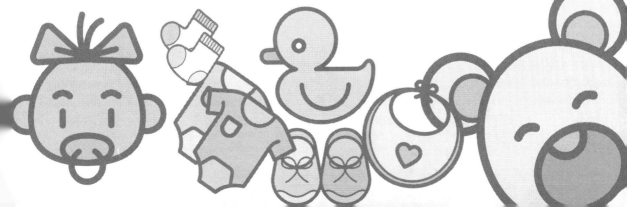

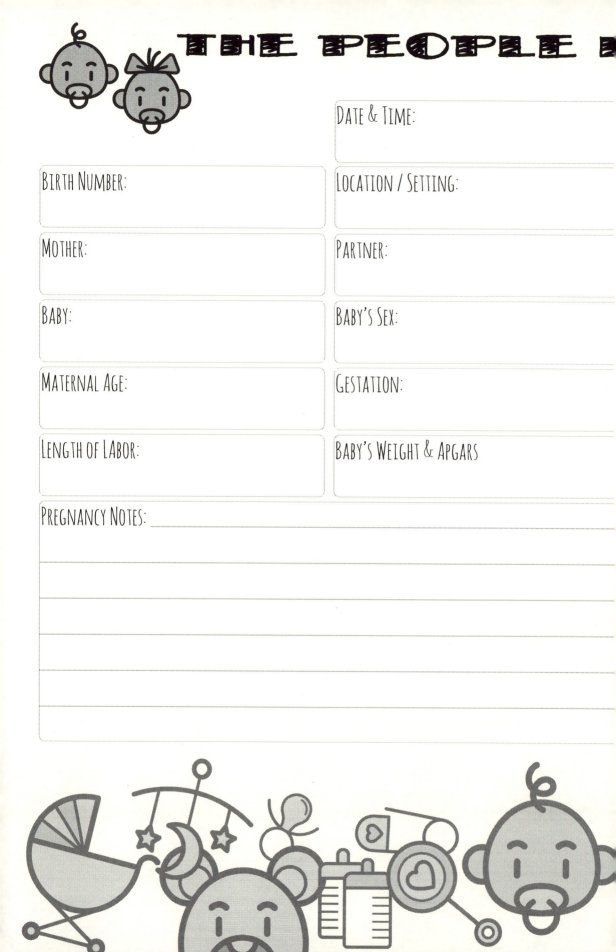

THE PEOPLE

Date & Time:

Birth Number:

Location / Setting:

Mother:

Partner:

Baby:

Baby's Sex:

Maternal Age:

Gestation:

Length of Labor:

Baby's Weight & Apgars

Pregnancy Notes:

HAVE HELPED OUT

COMMENTS:

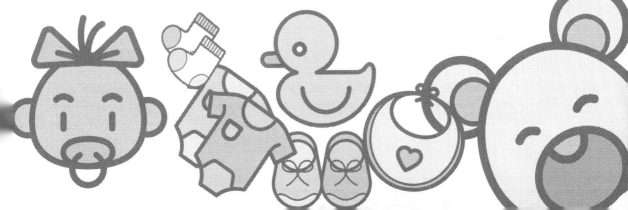

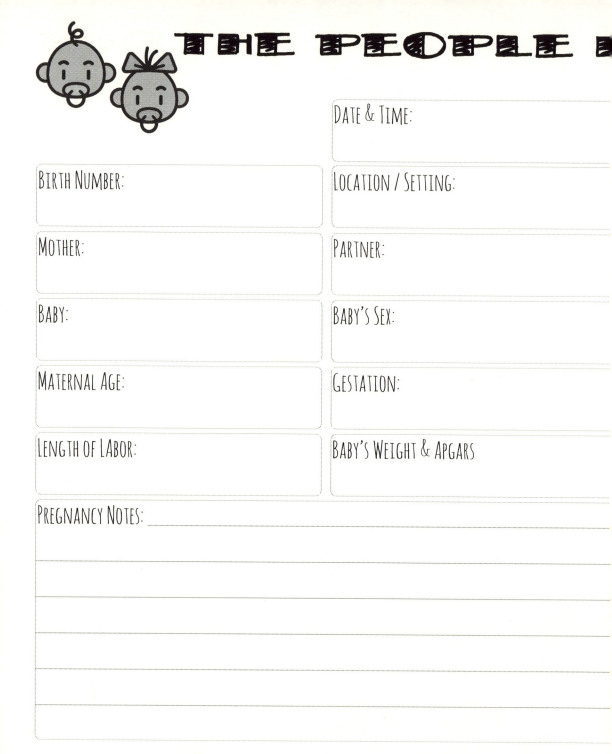

THE PEOPLE

Date & Time:

Birth Number:

Location / Setting:

Mother:

Partner:

Baby:

Baby's Sex:

Maternal Age:

Gestation:

Length of Labor:

Baby's Weight & Apgars

Pregnancy Notes:

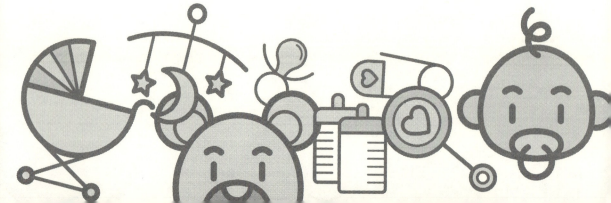

HAVE HELPED OUT

COMMENTS:

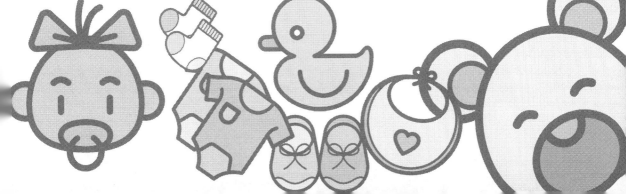

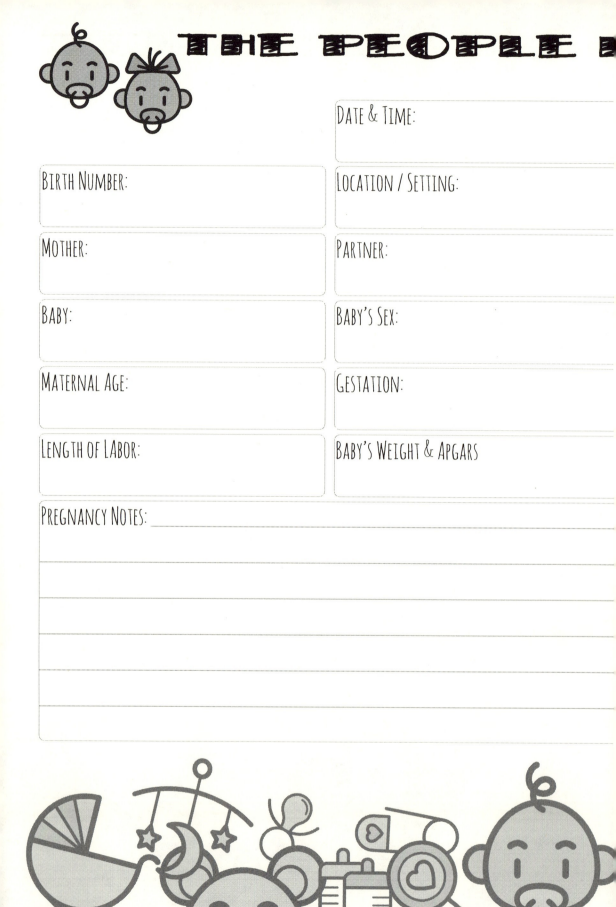

Date & Time:

Birth Number:

Location / Setting:

Mother:

Partner:

Baby:

Baby's Sex:

Maternal Age:

Gestation:

Length of Labor:

Baby's Weight & Apgars

Pregnancy Notes:

HAVE HELPED OUT

COMMENTS:

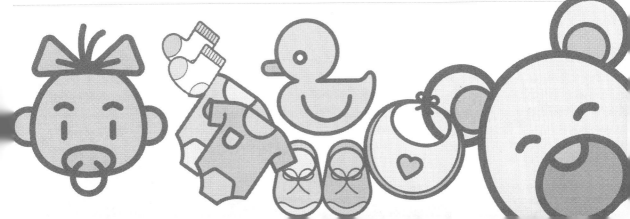

THE PEOPLE

Date & Time:

Birth Number:

Location / Setting:

Mother:

Partner:

Baby:

Baby's Sex:

Maternal Age:

Gestation:

Length of Labor:

Baby's Weight & Apgars

Pregnancy Notes:

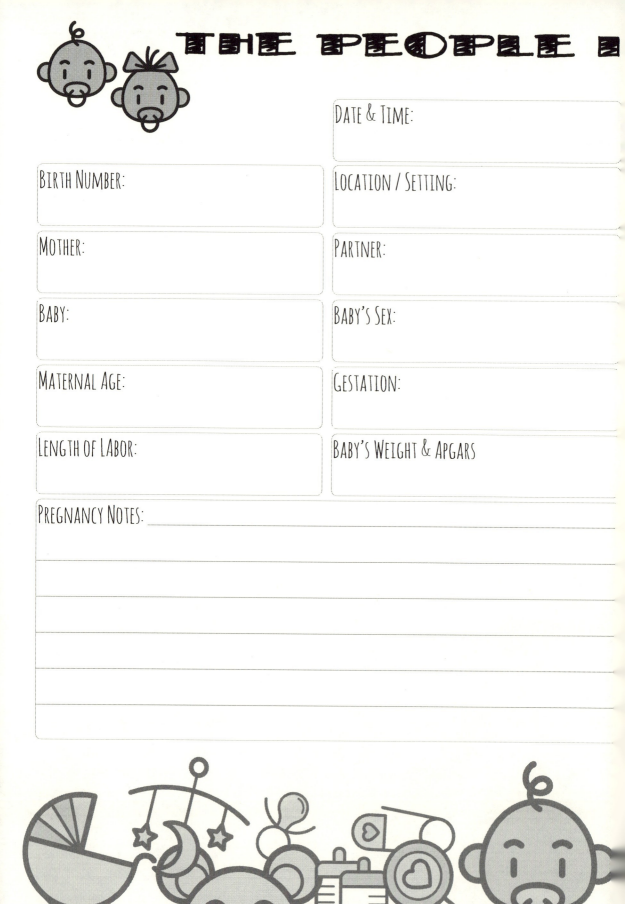

HAVE HELPED OUT

COMMENTS:

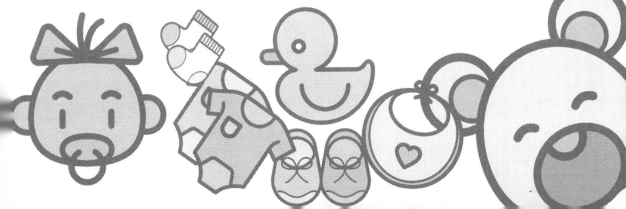

THE PEOPLE

Date & Time:

Birth Number:

Location / Setting:

Mother:

Partner:

Baby:

Baby's Sex:

Maternal Age:

Gestation:

Length of Labor:

Baby's Weight & Apgars

Pregnancy Notes:

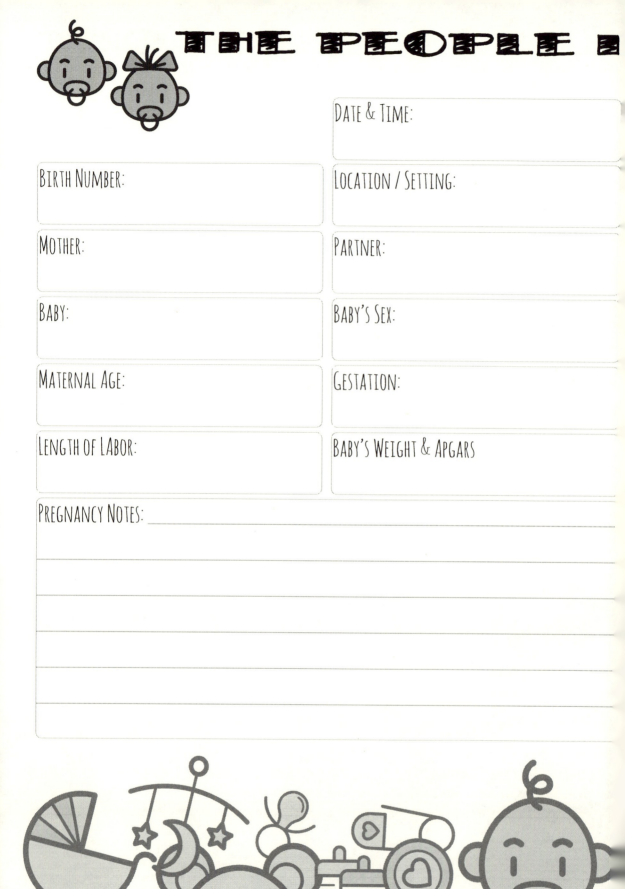

HAVE HELPED OUT

COMMENTS:

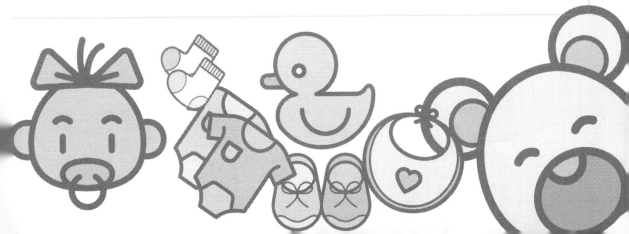

THE PEOPLE

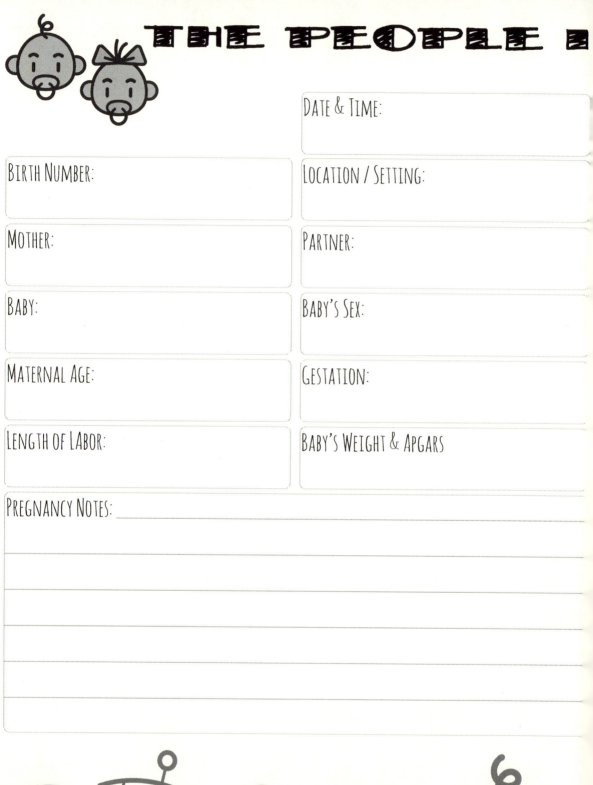

Date & Time:

Birth Number:

Location / Setting:

Mother:

Partner:

Baby:

Baby's Sex:

Maternal Age:

Gestation:

Length of Labor:

Baby's Weight & Apgars

Pregnancy Notes:

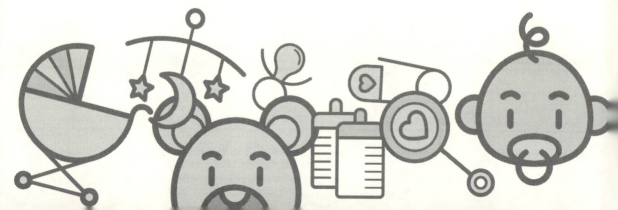

HAVE HELPED OUT

COMMENTS:

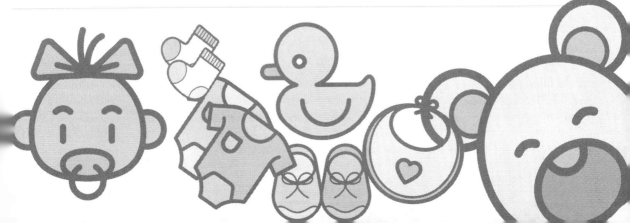

THE PEOPLE

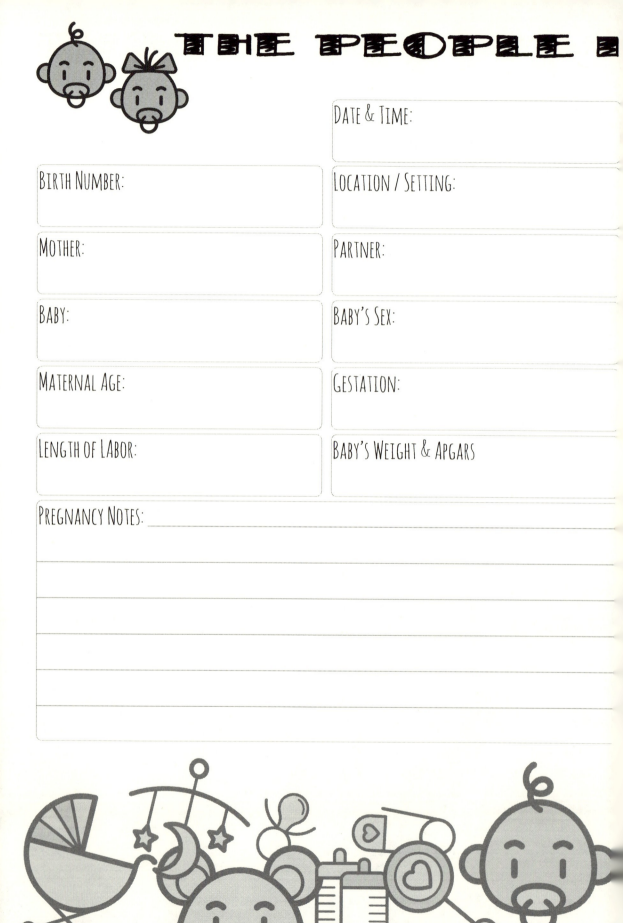

Date & Time:

Birth Number:

Location / Setting:

Mother:

Partner:

Baby:

Baby's Sex:

Maternal Age:

Gestation:

Length of Labor:

Baby's Weight & Apgars

Pregnancy Notes:

HAVE HELPED OUT

COMMENTS:

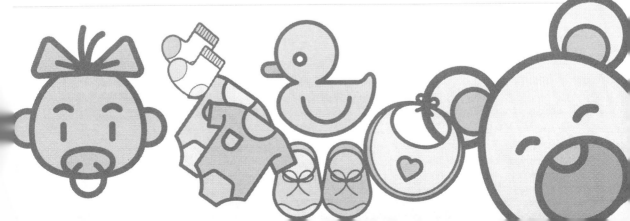

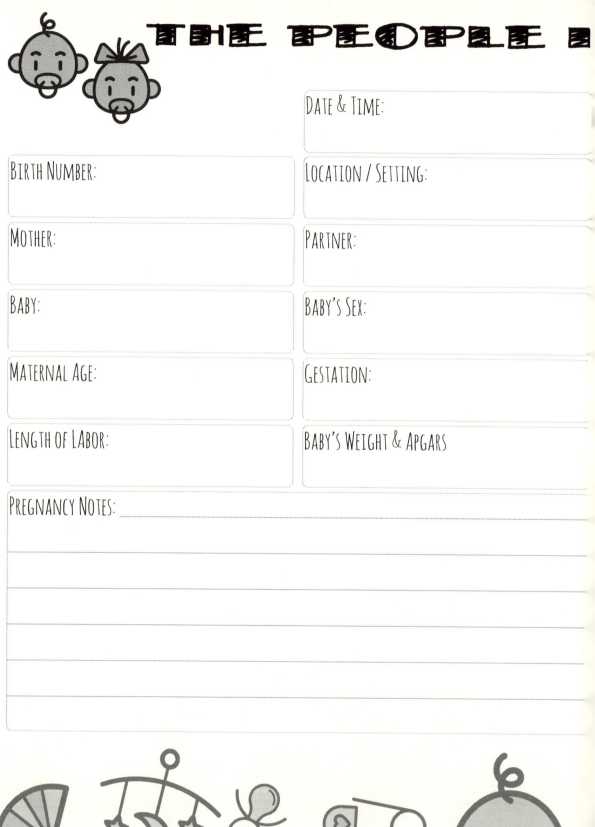

THE PEOPLE

Date & Time:

Birth Number:

Location / Setting:

Mother:

Partner:

Baby:

Baby's Sex:

Maternal Age:

Gestation:

Length of Labor:

Baby's Weight & Apgars

Pregnancy Notes:

HAVE HELPED OUT

COMMENTS:

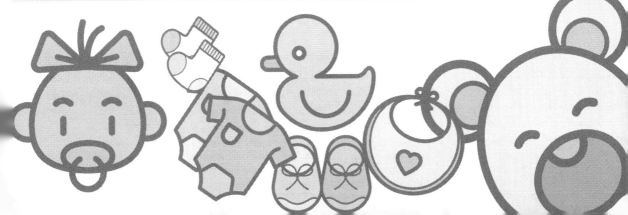

THE PEOPLE

Date & Time:

Birth Number:

Location / Setting:

Mother:

Partner:

Baby:

Baby's Sex:

Maternal Age:

Gestation:

Length of Labor:

Baby's Weight & Apgars

Pregnancy Notes:

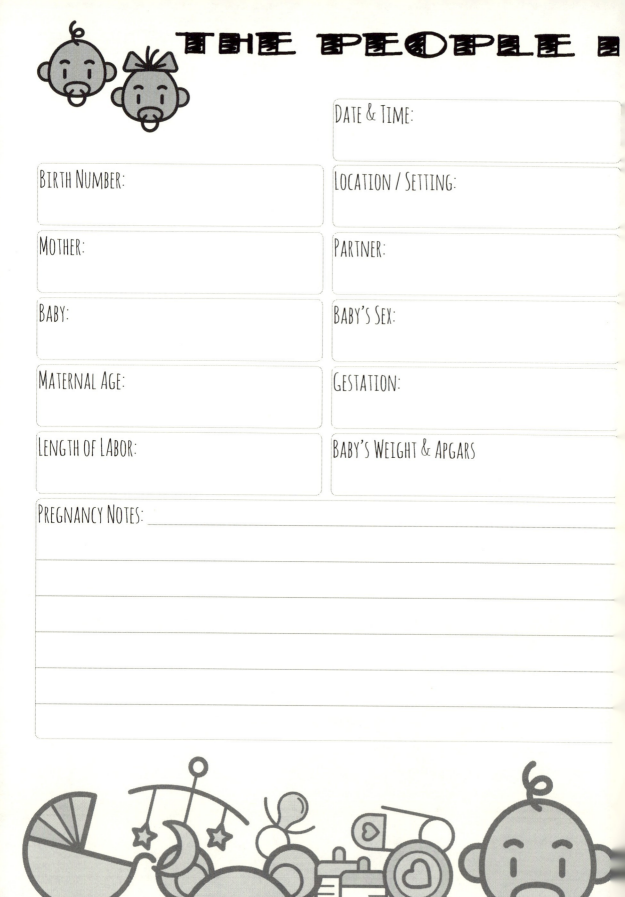

HAVE HELPED OUT

COMMENTS:

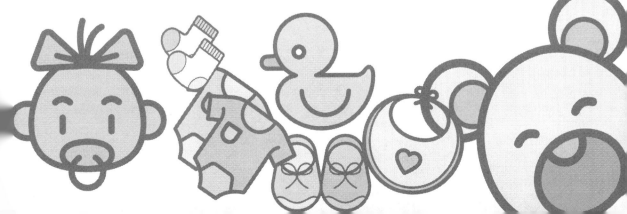

THE PEOPLE

Date & Time:

Birth Number:

Location / Setting:

Mother:

Partner:

Baby:

Baby's Sex:

Maternal Age:

Gestation:

Length of Labor:

Baby's Weight & Apgars

Pregnancy Notes:

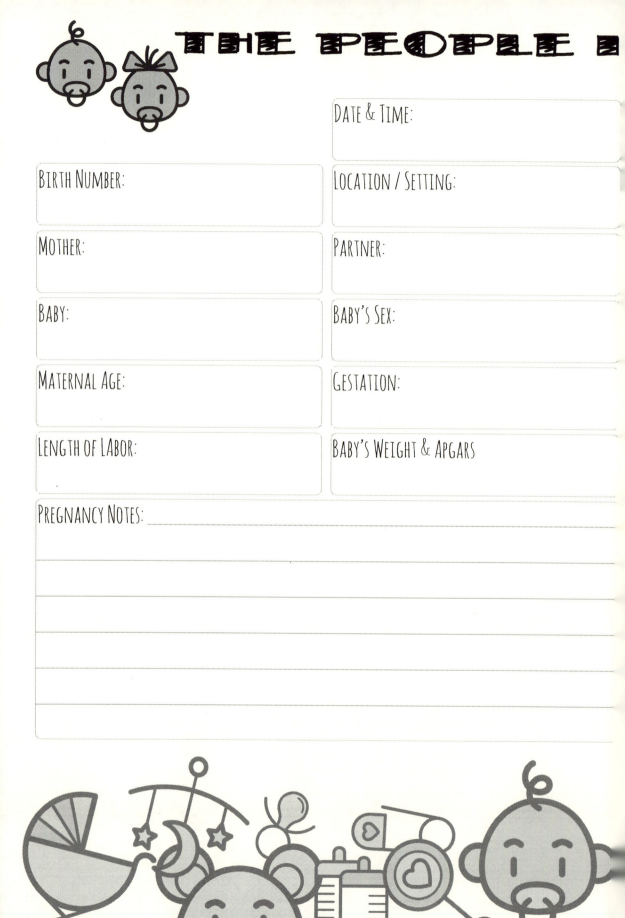

HAVE HELPED OUT

COMMENTS:

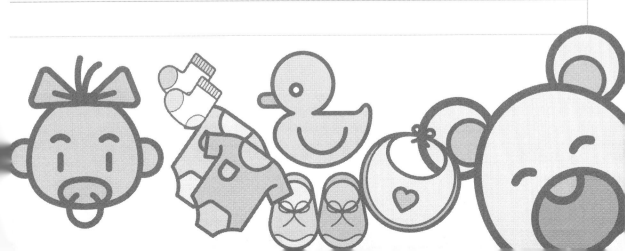

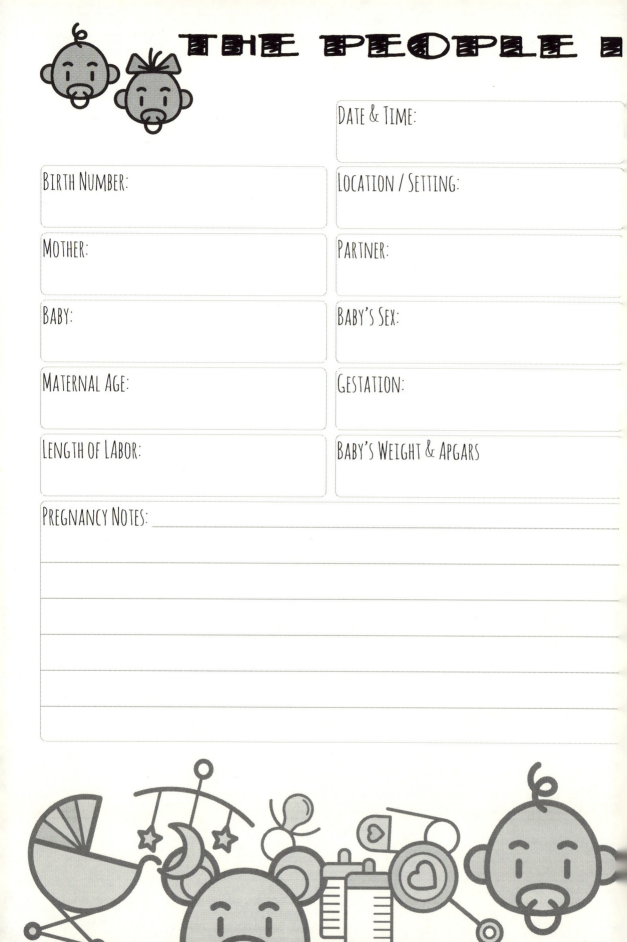

THE PEOPLE

Date & Time:

Birth Number:

Location / Setting:

Mother:

Partner:

Baby:

Baby's Sex:

Maternal Age:

Gestation:

Length of Labor:

Baby's Weight & Apgars

Pregnancy Notes:

HAVE HELPED OUT

COMMENTS:

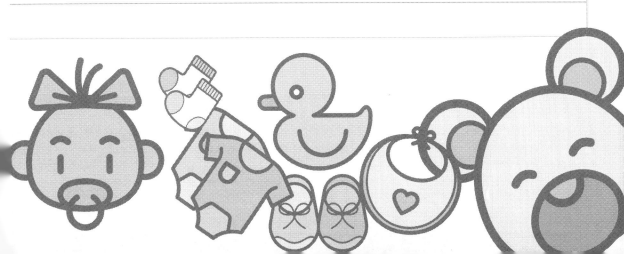

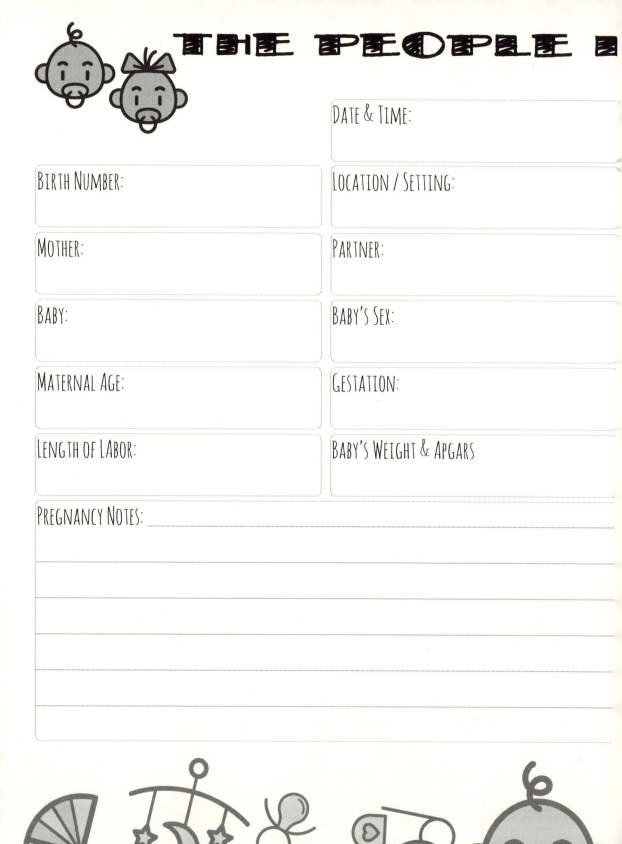

THE PEOPLE

Date & Time:

Birth Number:

Location / Setting:

Mother:

Partner:

Baby:

Baby's Sex:

Maternal Age:

Gestation:

Length of Labor:

Baby's Weight & Apgars

Pregnancy Notes:

HAVE HELPED OUT

COMMENTS:

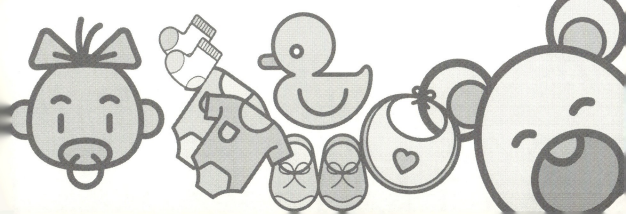

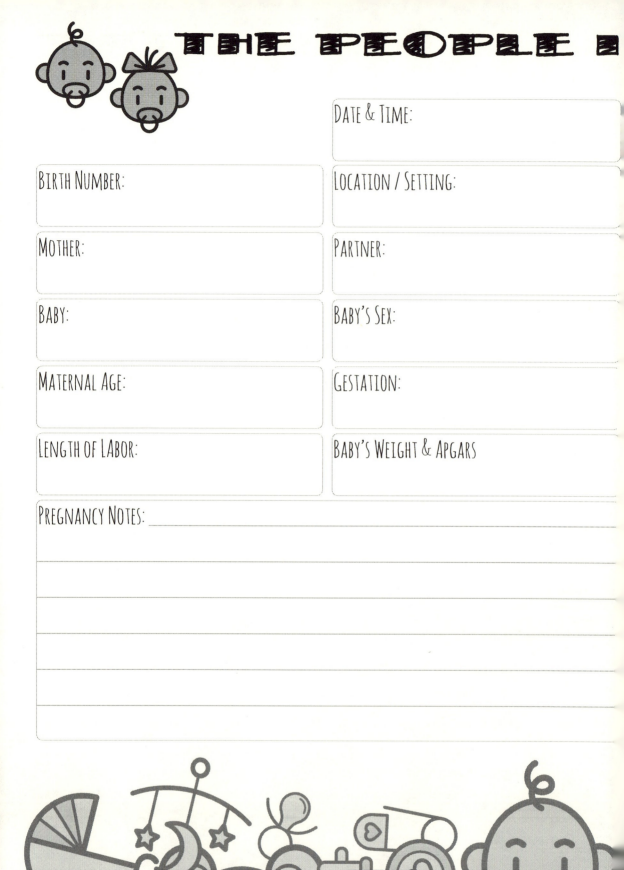

THE PEOPLE

Date & Time:

Birth Number:

Location / Setting:

Mother:

Partner:

Baby:

Baby's Sex:

Maternal Age:

Gestation:

Length of Labor:

Baby's Weight & Apgars

Pregnancy Notes:

HAVE HELPED OUT

COMMENTS:

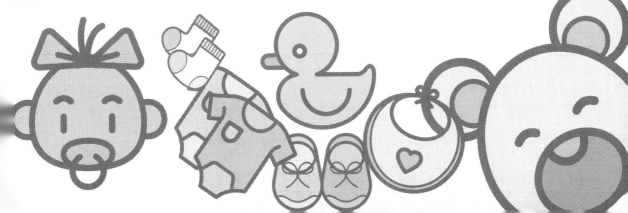

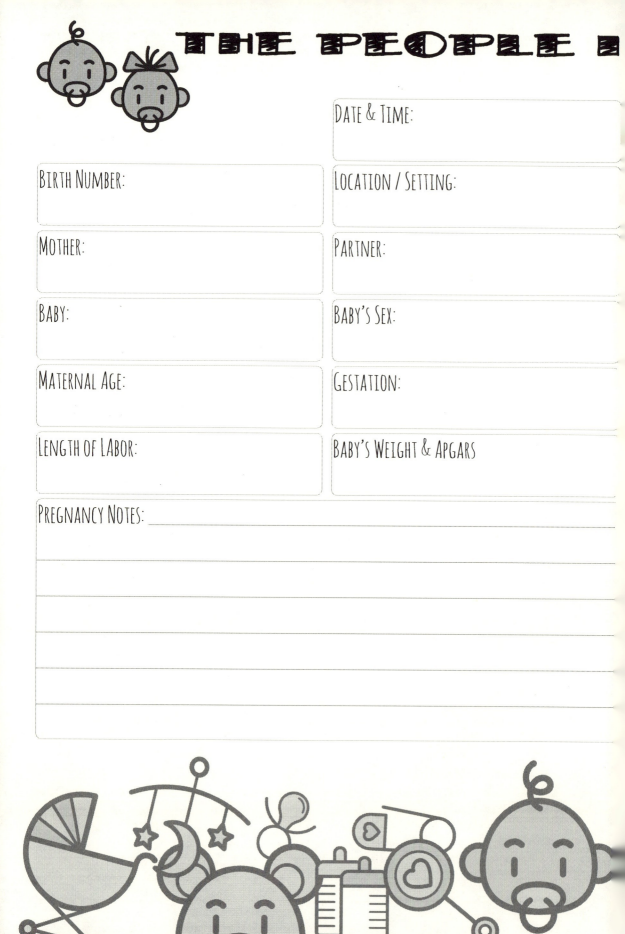

THE PEOPLE

DATE & TIME:

BIRTH NUMBER:

LOCATION / SETTING:

MOTHER:

PARTNER:

BABY:

BABY'S SEX:

MATERNAL AGE:

GESTATION:

LENGTH OF LABOR:

BABY'S WEIGHT & APGARS

PREGNANCY NOTES:

HAVE HELPED OUT

COMMENTS:

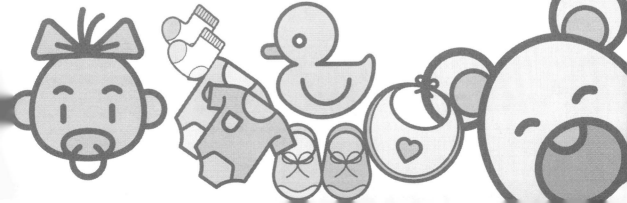

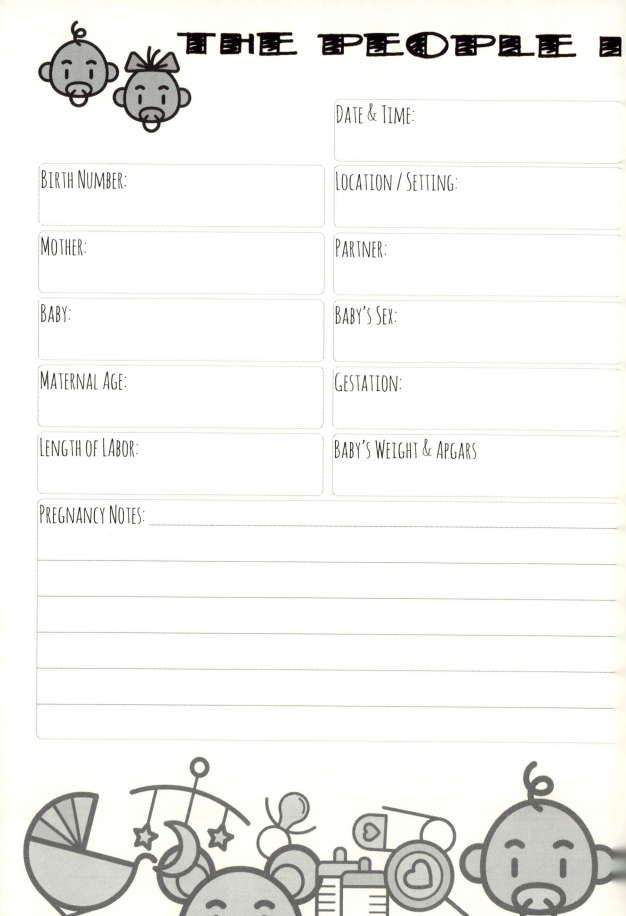

THE PEOPLE

Date & Time:

Birth Number:

Location / Setting:

Mother:

Partner:

Baby:

Baby's Sex:

Maternal Age:

Gestation:

Length of Labor:

Baby's Weight & Apgars

Pregnancy Notes:

HAVE HELPED OUT

COMMENTS:

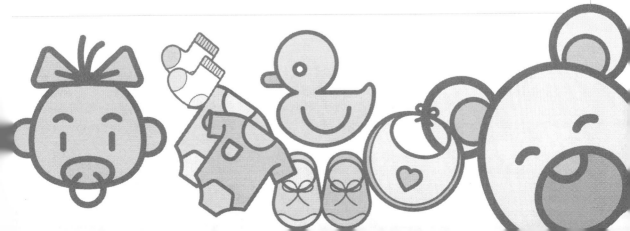

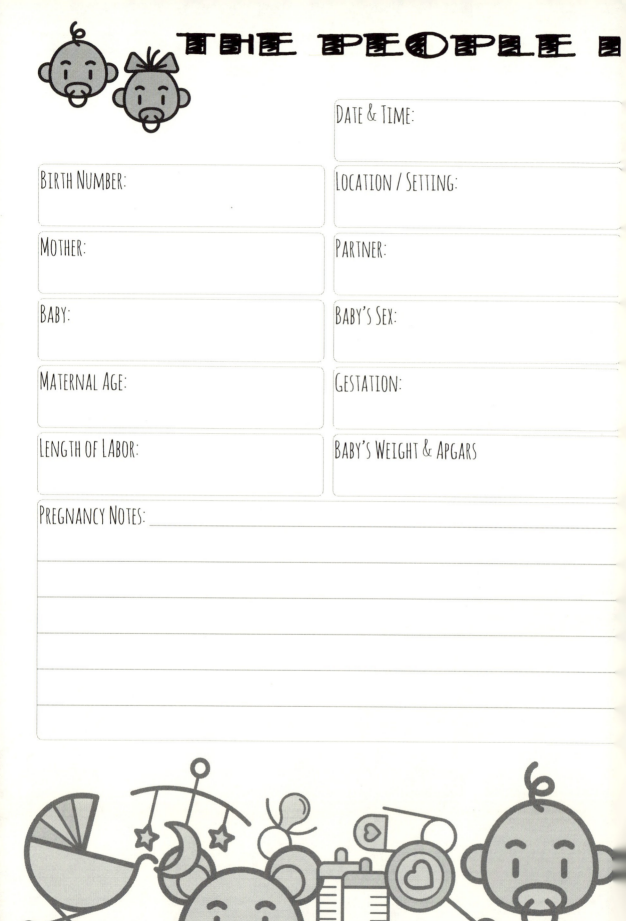

THE PEOPLE

Date & Time:

Birth Number:

Location / Setting:

Mother:

Partner:

Baby:

Baby's Sex:

Maternal Age:

Gestation:

Length of Labor:

Baby's Weight & Apgars

Pregnancy Notes:

HAVE HELPED OUT

COMMENTS:

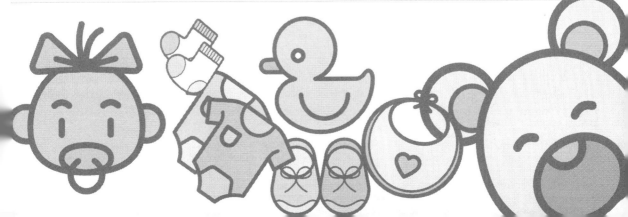

THE PEOPLE

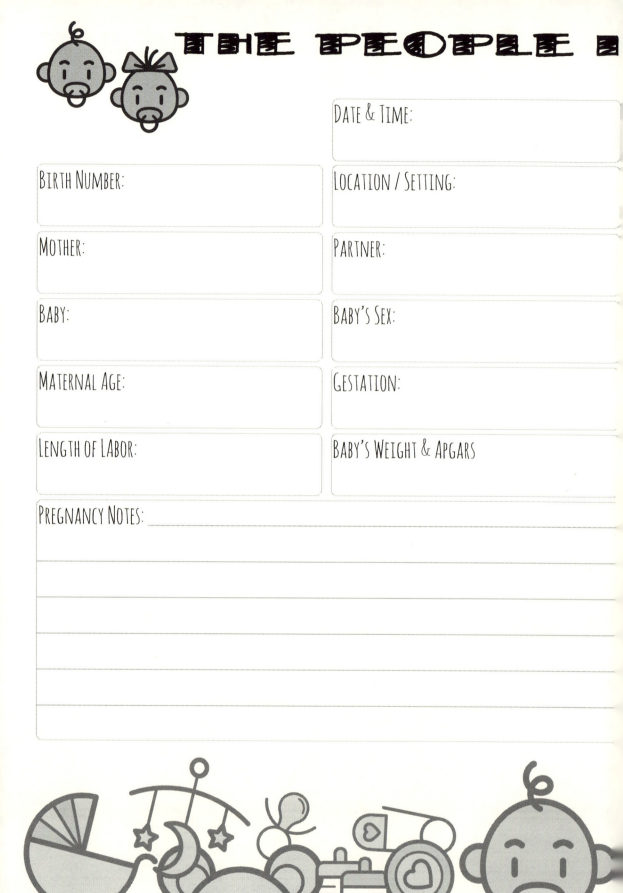

Date & Time:

Birth Number:

Location / Setting:

Mother:

Partner:

Baby:

Baby's Sex:

Maternal Age:

Gestation:

Length of Labor:

Baby's Weight & Apgars

Pregnancy Notes:

HAVE HELPED OUT

COMMENTS:

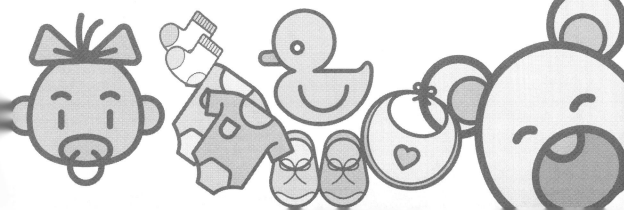

THE PEOPLE

Date & Time:

Birth Number:

Location / Setting:

Mother:

Partner:

Baby:

Baby's Sex:

Maternal Age:

Gestation:

Length of Labor:

Baby's Weight & Apgars

Pregnancy Notes:

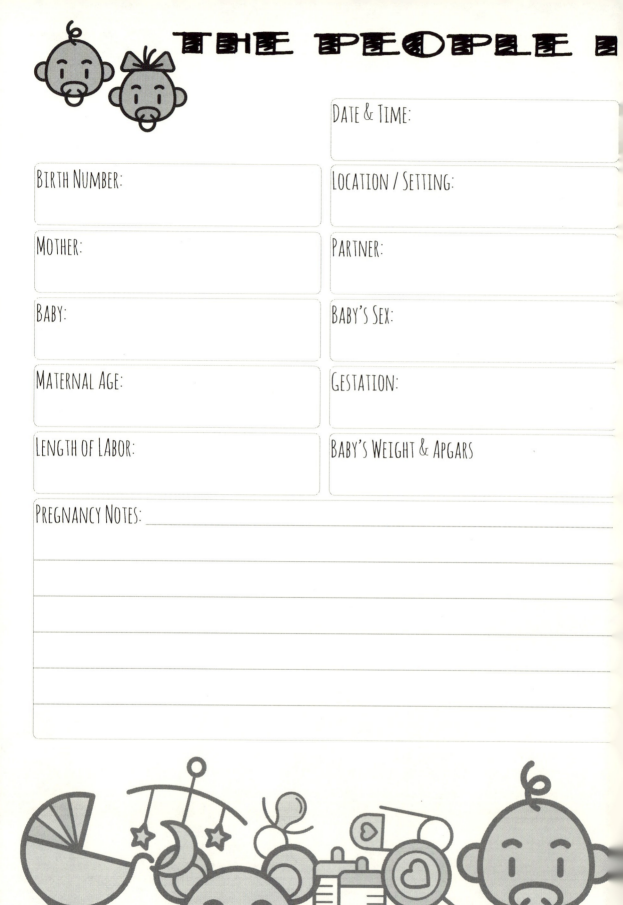

HAVE HELPED OUT

COMMENTS:

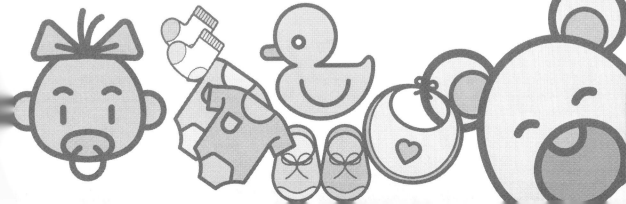

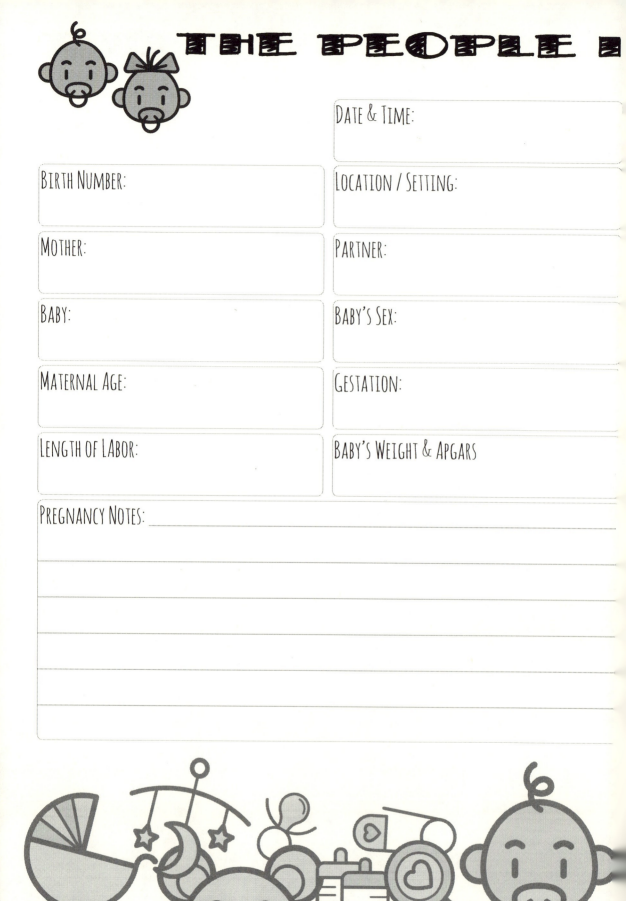

THE PEOPLE

Date & Time:

Birth Number:

Location / Setting:

Mother:

Partner:

Baby:

Baby's Sex:

Maternal Age:

Gestation:

Length of Labor:

Baby's Weight & Apgars

Pregnancy Notes:

HAVE HELPED OUT

COMMENTS:

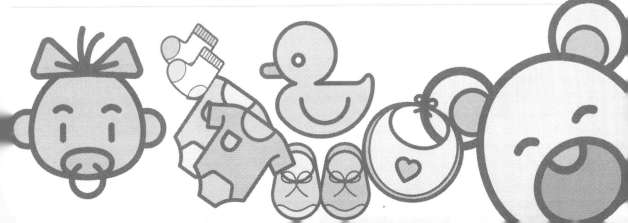

THE PEOPLE

Date & Time:

Birth Number:

Location / Setting:

Mother:

Partner:

Baby:

Baby's Sex:

Maternal Age:

Gestation:

Length of Labor:

Baby's Weight & Apgars

Pregnancy Notes:

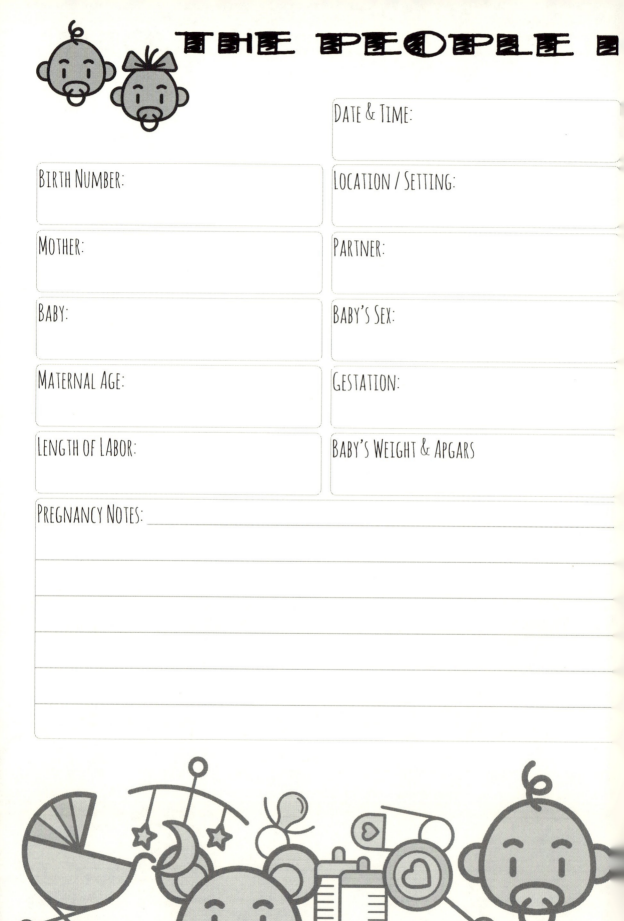

HAVE HELPED OUT

COMMENTS:

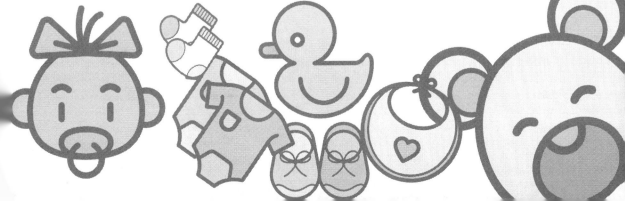

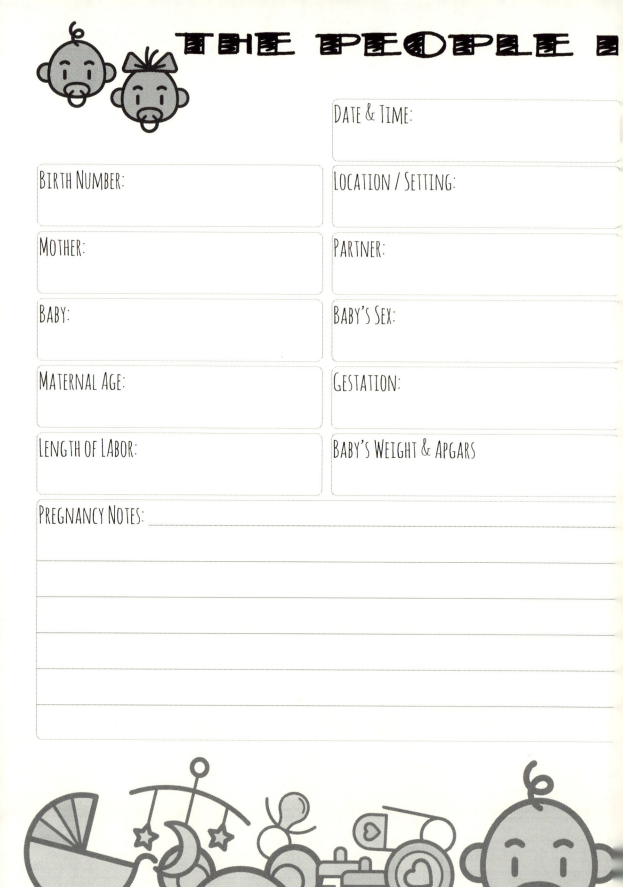

THE PEOPLE &

Date & Time:

Birth Number:

Location / Setting:

Mother:

Partner:

Baby:

Baby's Sex:

Maternal Age:

Gestation:

Length of Labor:

Baby's Weight & Apgars

Pregnancy Notes:

HAVE HELPED OUT

COMMENTS:

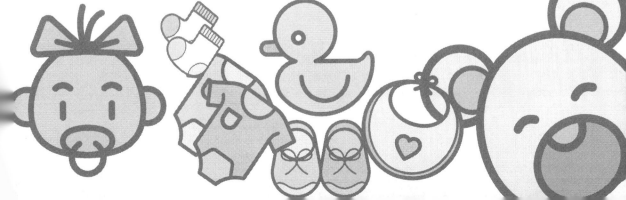

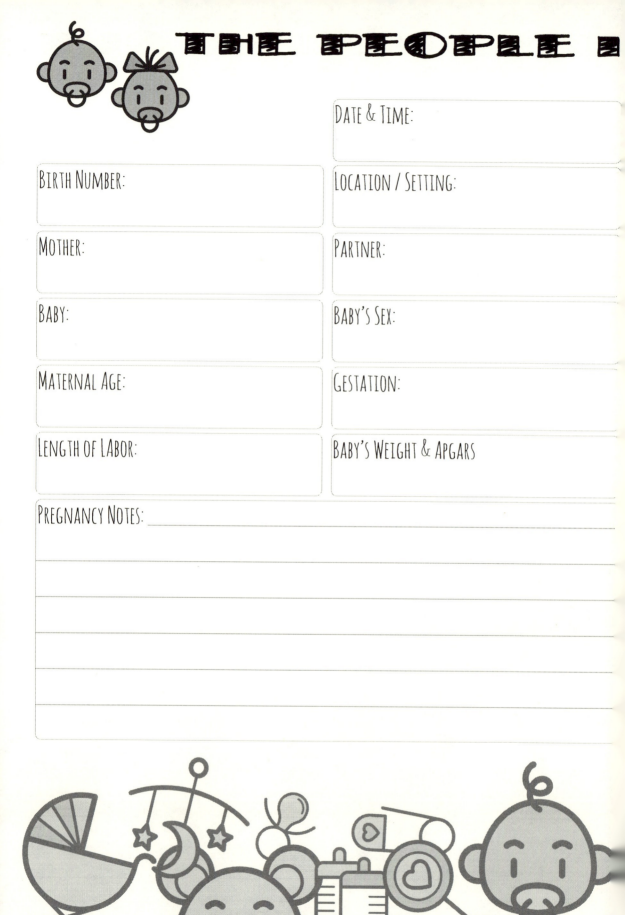

THE PEOPLE

Date & Time:

Birth Number:

Location / Setting:

Mother:

Partner:

Baby:

Baby's Sex:

Maternal Age:

Gestation:

Length of Labor:

Baby's Weight & Apgars

Pregnancy Notes:

HAVE HELPED OUT

COMMENTS:

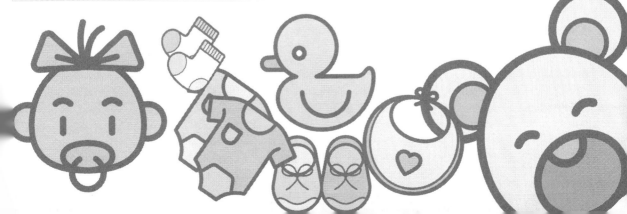

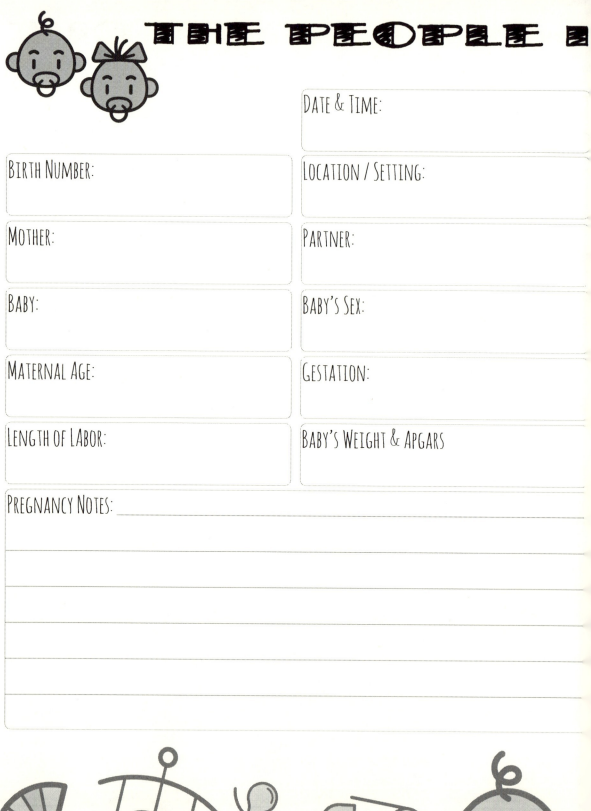

THE PEOPLE

Date & Time:

Birth Number:

Location / Setting:

Mother:

Partner:

Baby:

Baby's Sex:

Maternal Age:

Gestation:

Length of Labor:

Baby's Weight & Apgars

Pregnancy Notes:

HAVE HELPED OUT

COMMENTS:

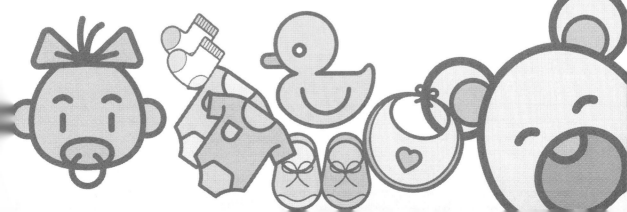

THE PEOPLE

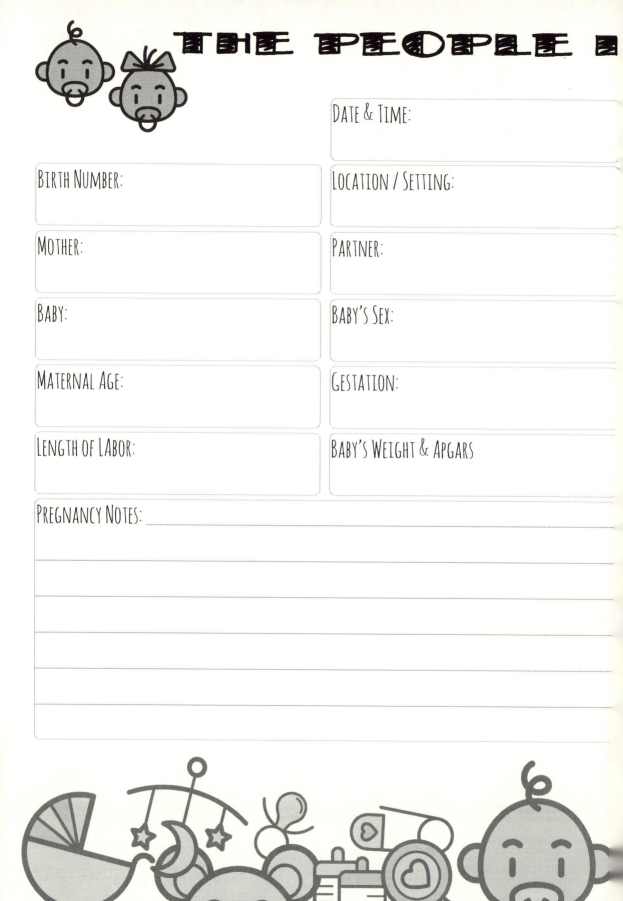

Date & Time:

Birth Number:

Location / Setting:

Mother:

Partner:

Baby:

Baby's Sex:

Maternal Age:

Gestation:

Length of Labor:

Baby's Weight & Apgars

Pregnancy Notes:

HAVE HELPED OUT

COMMENTS:

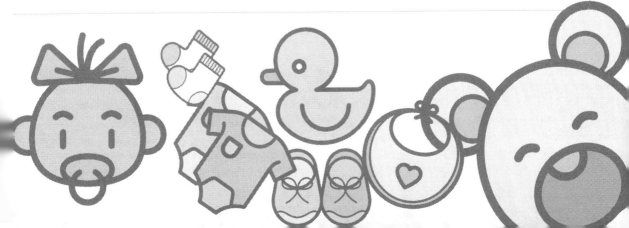

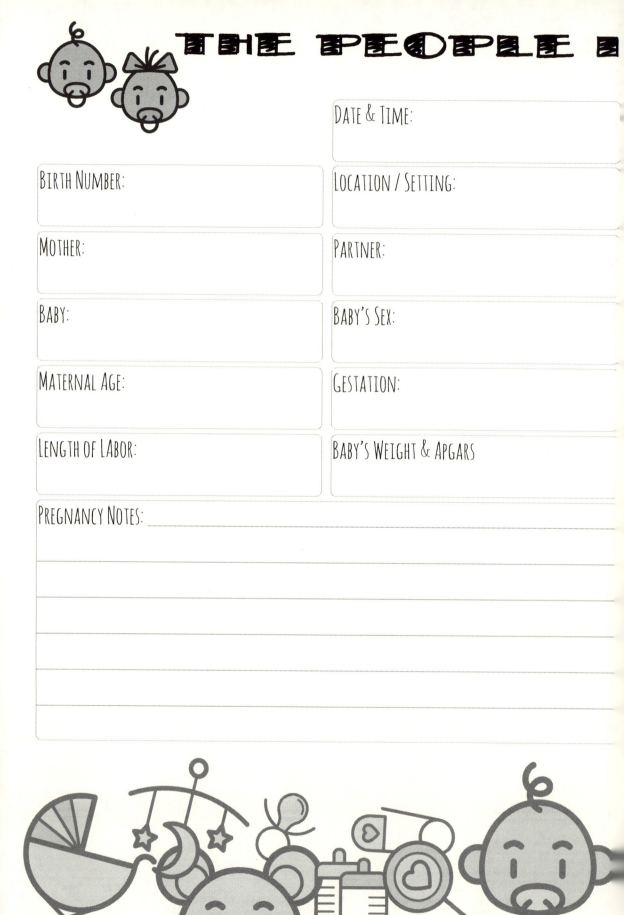

THE PEOPLE

Date & Time:

Birth Number:

Location / Setting:

Mother:

Partner:

Baby:

Baby's Sex:

Maternal Age:

Gestation:

Length of Labor:

Baby's Weight & Apgars

Pregnancy Notes:

HAVE HELPED OUT

COMMENTS:

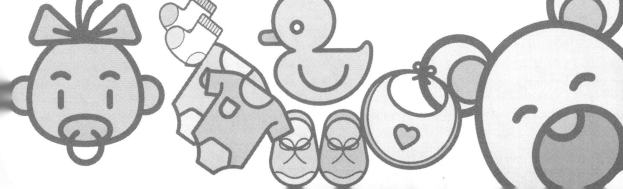

THE PEOPLE

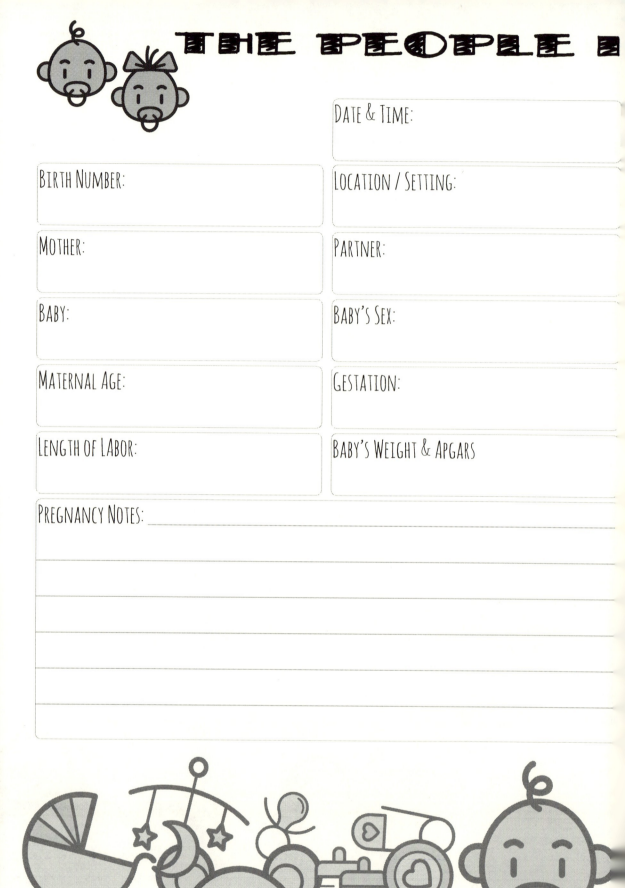

DATE & TIME:

BIRTH NUMBER:

LOCATION / SETTING:

MOTHER:

PARTNER:

BABY:

BABY'S SEX:

MATERNAL AGE:

GESTATION:

LENGTH OF LABOR:

BABY'S WEIGHT & APGARS

PREGNANCY NOTES:

HAVE HELPED OUT

COMMENTS:

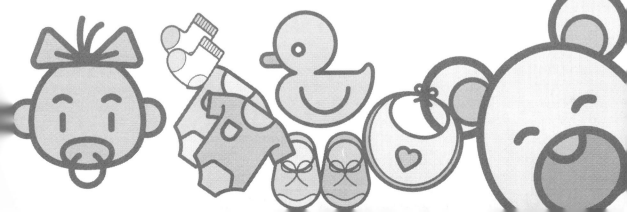

THE PEOPLE

Date & Time:

Birth Number:

Location / Setting:

Mother:

Partner:

Baby:

Baby's Sex:

Maternal Age:

Gestation:

Length of Labor:

Baby's Weight & Apgars

Pregnancy Notes:

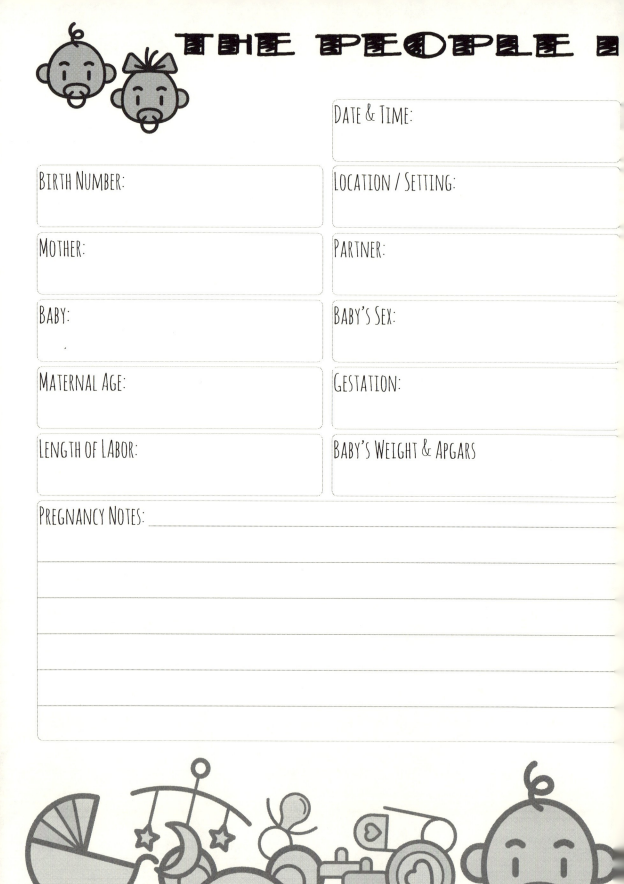

HAVE HELPED OUT

COMMENTS:

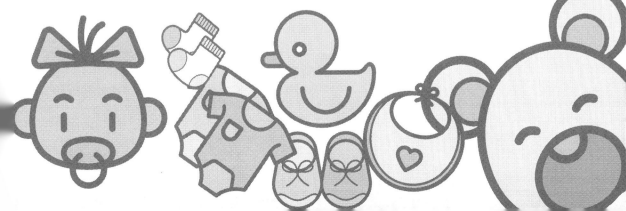

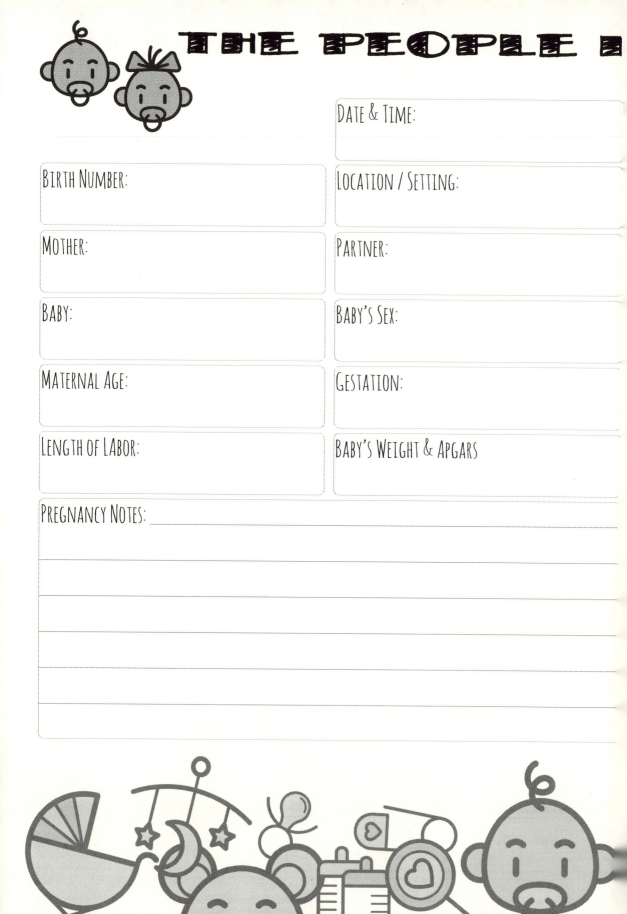

THE PEOPLE

DATE & TIME:

BIRTH NUMBER:

LOCATION / SETTING:

MOTHER:

PARTNER:

BABY:

BABY'S SEX:

MATERNAL AGE:

GESTATION:

LENGTH OF LABOR:

BABY'S WEIGHT & APGARS

PREGNANCY NOTES:

HAVE HELPED OUT

COMMENTS:

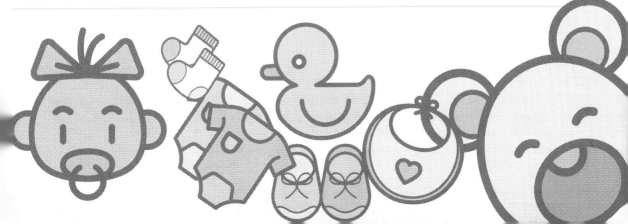

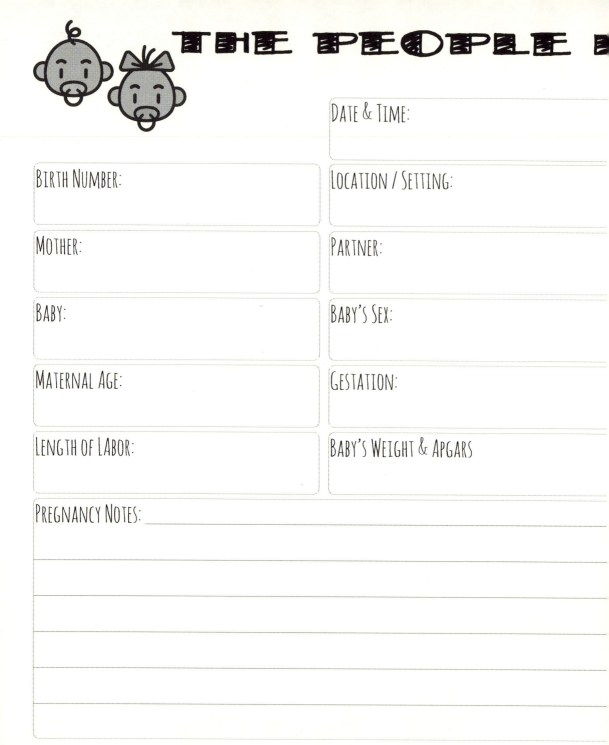

THE PEOPLE

Date & Time:

Birth Number:

Location / Setting:

Mother:

Partner:

Baby:

Baby's Sex:

Maternal Age:

Gestation:

Length of Labor:

Baby's Weight & Apgars

Pregnancy Notes:

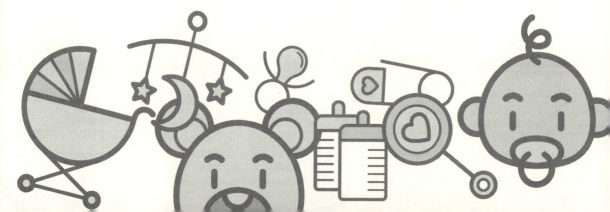

HAVE HELPED OUT

COMMENTS:

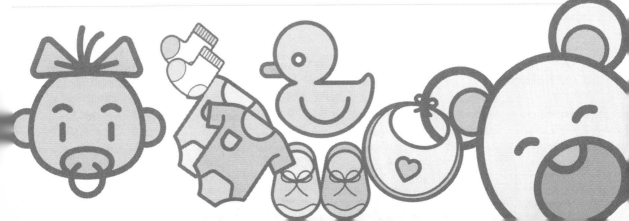

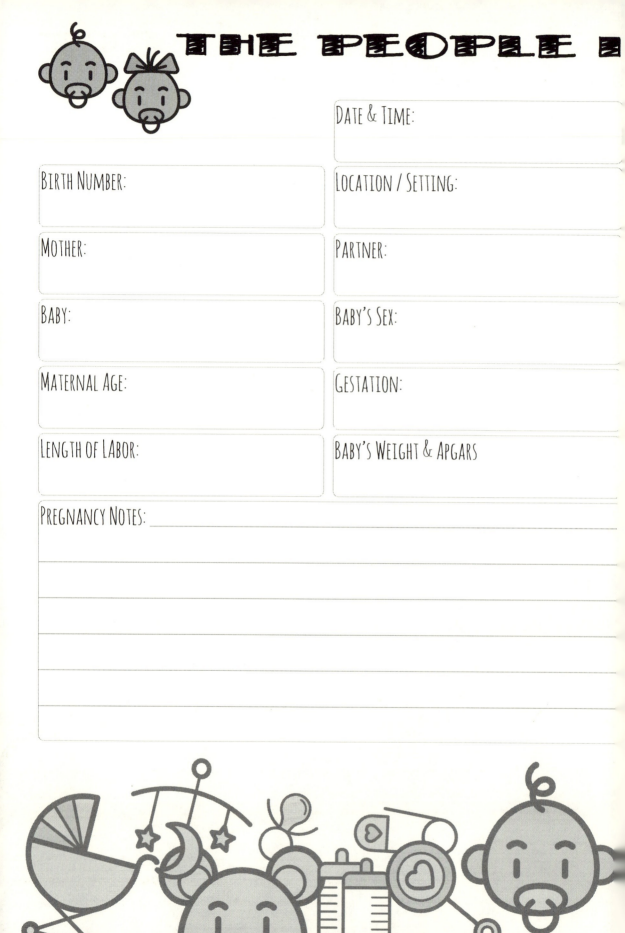

THE PEOPLE

Date & Time:

Birth Number:

Location / Setting:

Mother:

Partner:

Baby:

Baby's Sex:

Maternal Age:

Gestation:

Length of Labor:

Baby's Weight & Apgars

Pregnancy Notes:

HAVE HELPED OUT

COMMENTS:

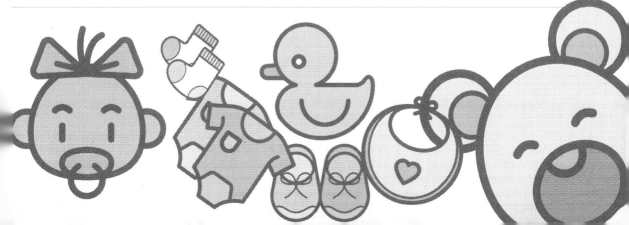

THE PEOPLE

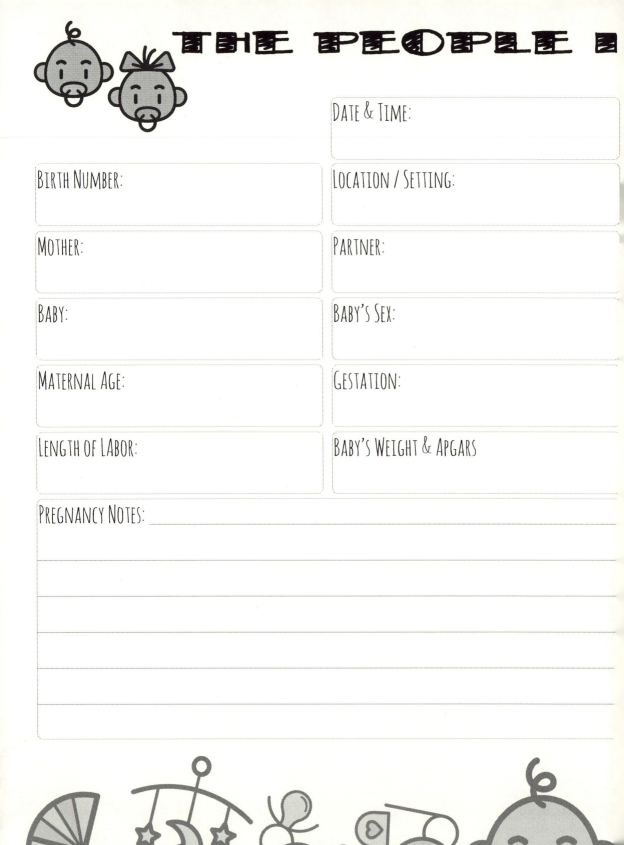

Date & Time:

Birth Number:

Location / Setting:

Mother:

Partner:

Baby:

Baby's Sex:

Maternal Age:

Gestation:

Length of Labor:

Baby's Weight & Apgars

Pregnancy Notes:

HAVE HELPED OUT

COMMENTS:

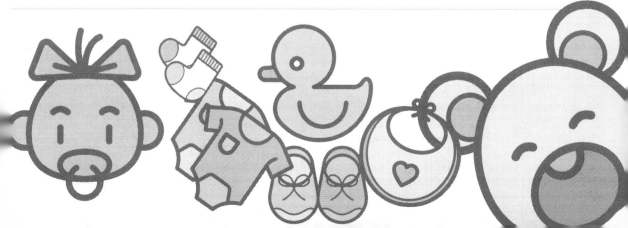

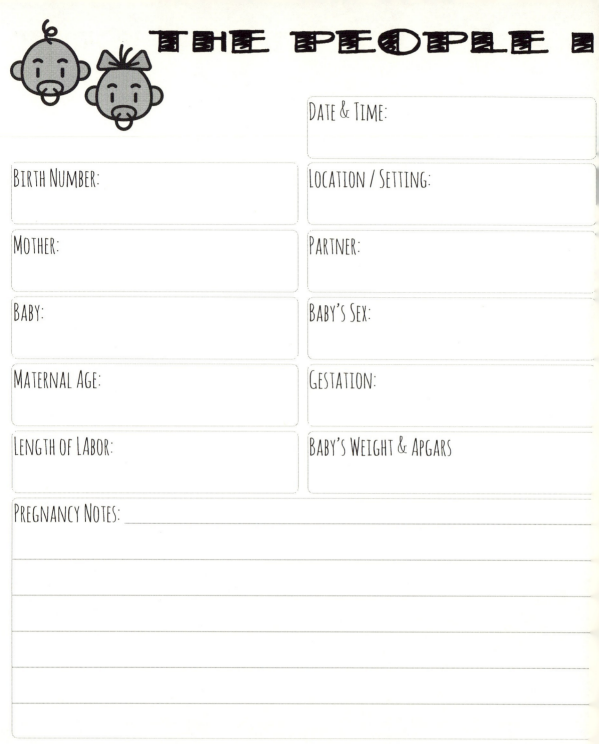

THE PEOPLE

Date & Time:

Birth Number:

Location / Setting:

Mother:

Partner:

Baby:

Baby's Sex:

Maternal Age:

Gestation:

Length of Labor:

Baby's Weight & Apgars

Pregnancy Notes:

HAVE HELPED OUT

COMMENTS:

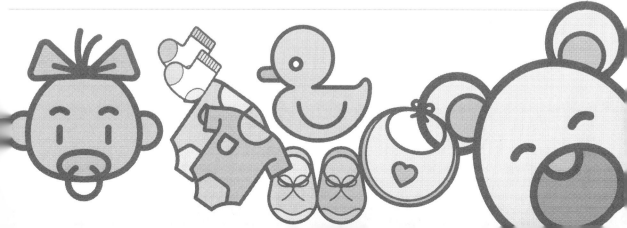

THE PEOPLE

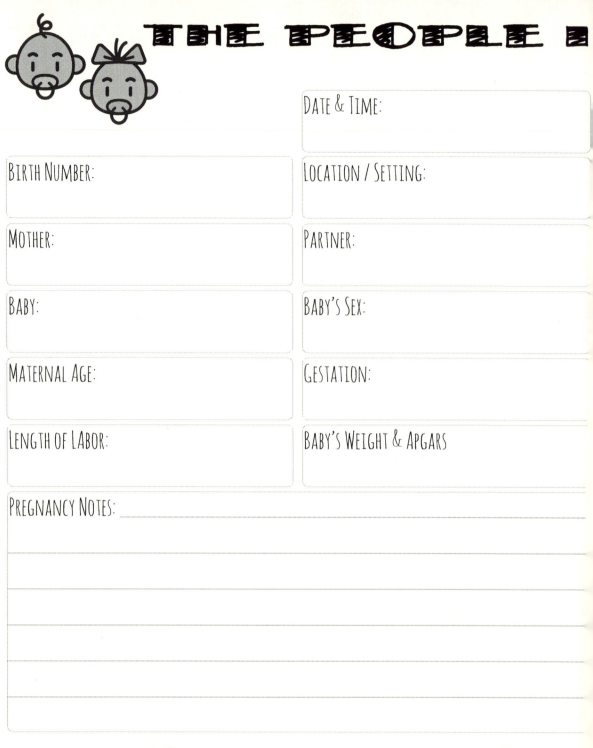

DATE & TIME:

BIRTH NUMBER:

LOCATION / SETTING:

MOTHER:

PARTNER:

BABY:

BABY'S SEX:

MATERNAL AGE:

GESTATION:

LENGTH OF LABOR:

BABY'S WEIGHT & APGARS

PREGNANCY NOTES:

HAVE HELPED OUT

COMMENTS:

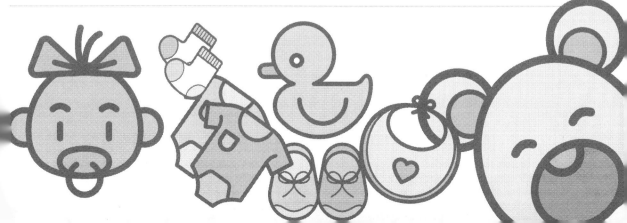

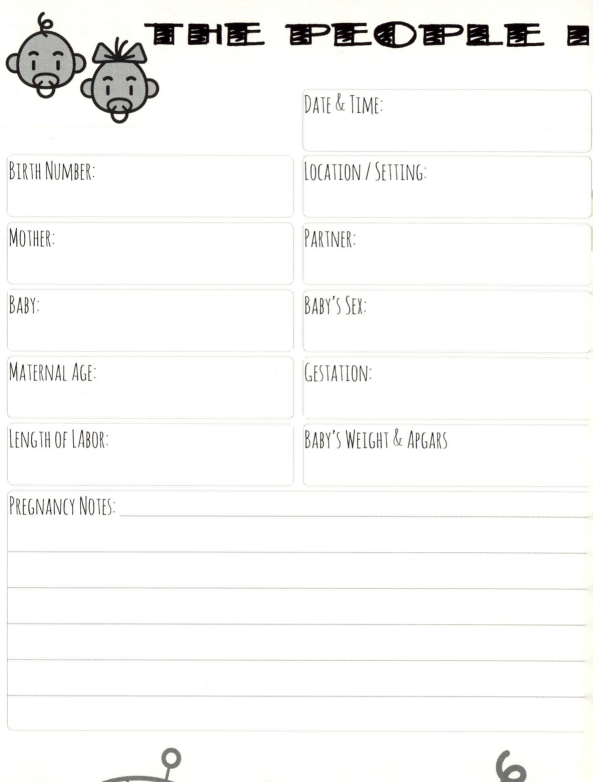

THE PEOPLE

Date & Time:

Birth Number:

Location / Setting:

Mother:

Partner:

Baby:

Baby's Sex:

Maternal Age:

Gestation:

Length of Labor:

Baby's Weight & Apgars

Pregnancy Notes:

HAVE HELPED OUT

COMMENTS:

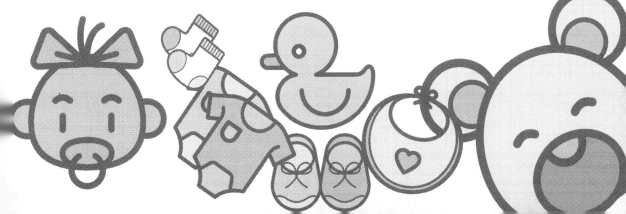

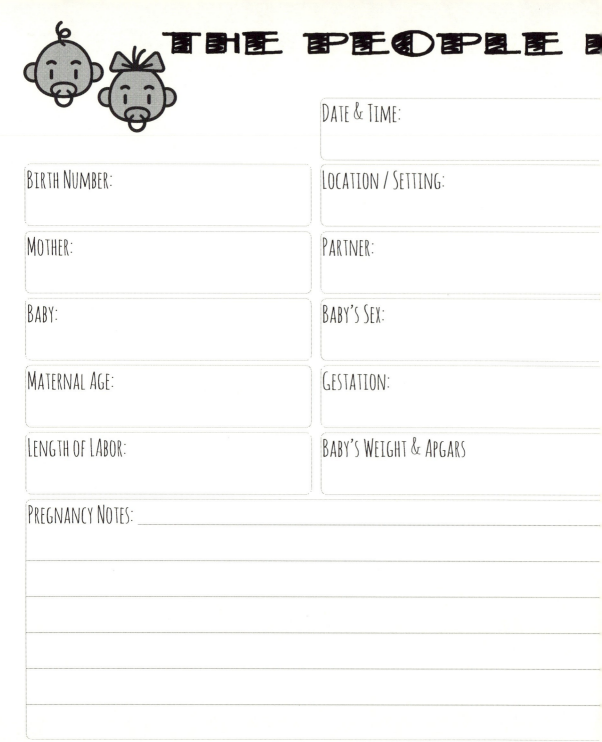

THE PEOPLE

Date & Time:

Birth Number:

Location / Setting:

Mother:

Partner:

Baby:

Baby's Sex:

Maternal Age:

Gestation:

Length of Labor:

Baby's Weight & Apgars

Pregnancy Notes:

HAVE HELPED OUT

COMMENTS:

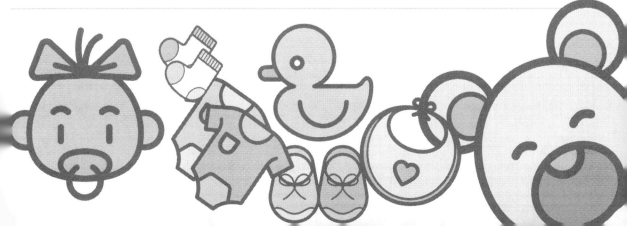

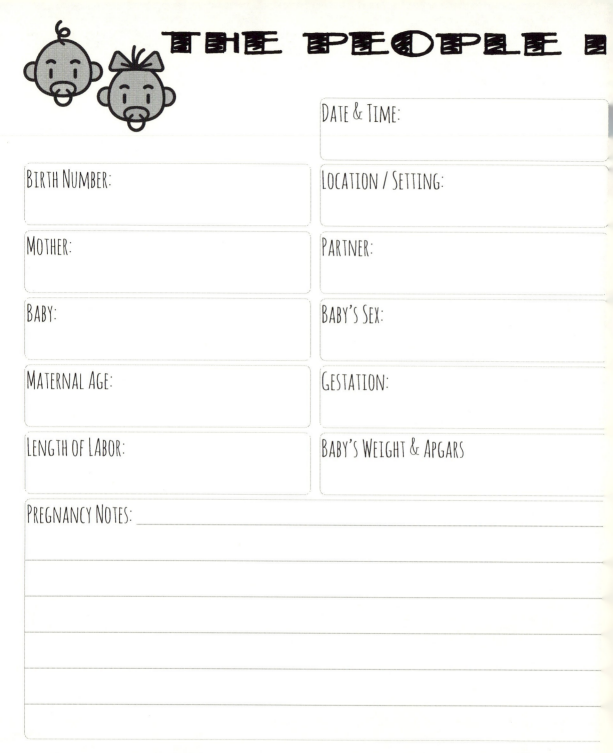

THE PEOPLE

Date & Time:

Birth Number:

Location / Setting:

Mother:

Partner:

Baby:

Baby's Sex:

Maternal Age:

Gestation:

Length of Labor:

Baby's Weight & Apgars

Pregnancy Notes:

HAVE HELPED OUT

COMMENTS:

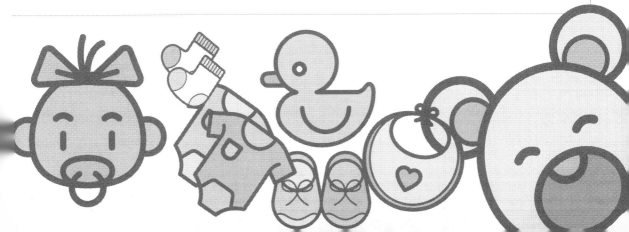

THE PEOPLE

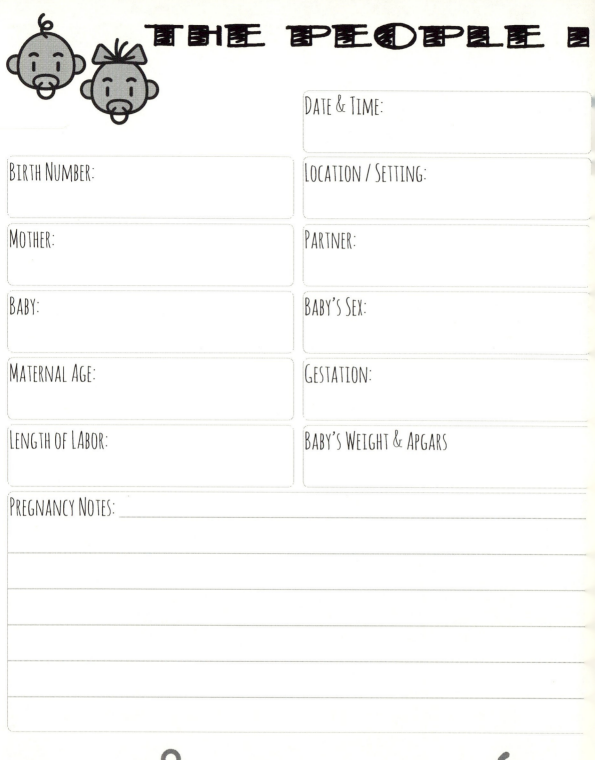

Date & Time:

Birth Number:

Location / Setting:

Mother:

Partner:

Baby:

Baby's Sex:

Maternal Age:

Gestation:

Length of Labor:

Baby's Weight & Apgars

Pregnancy Notes:

HAVE HELPED OUT

COMMENTS:

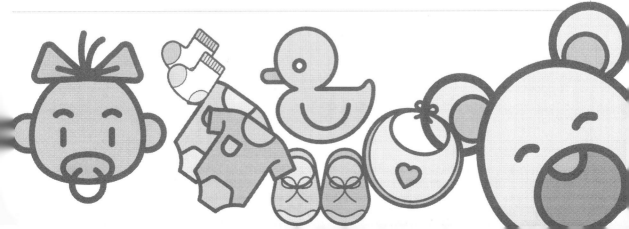

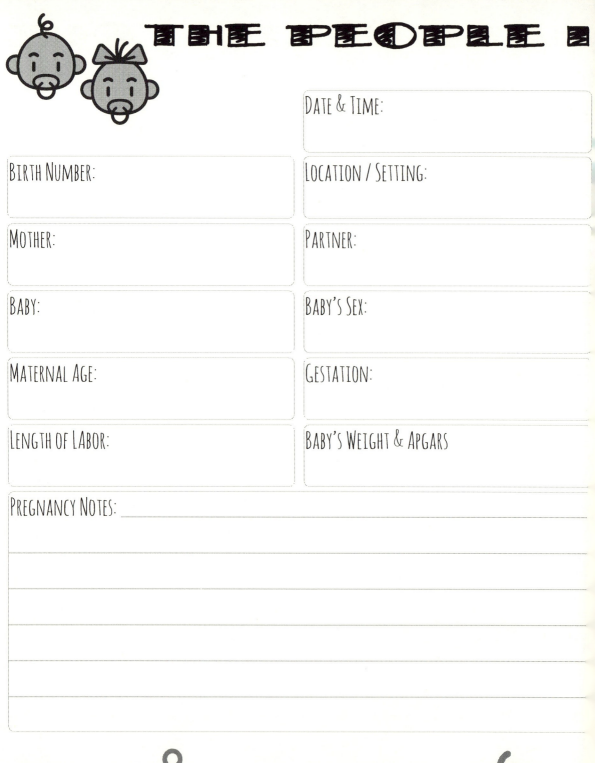

THE PEOPLE

Date & Time:

Birth Number:

Location / Setting:

Mother:

Partner:

Baby:

Baby's Sex:

Maternal Age:

Gestation:

Length of Labor:

Baby's Weight & Apgars

Pregnancy Notes:

HAVE HELPED OUT

COMMENTS:

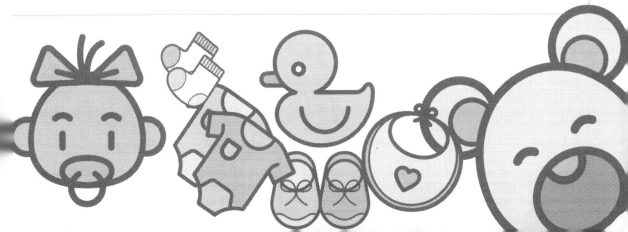

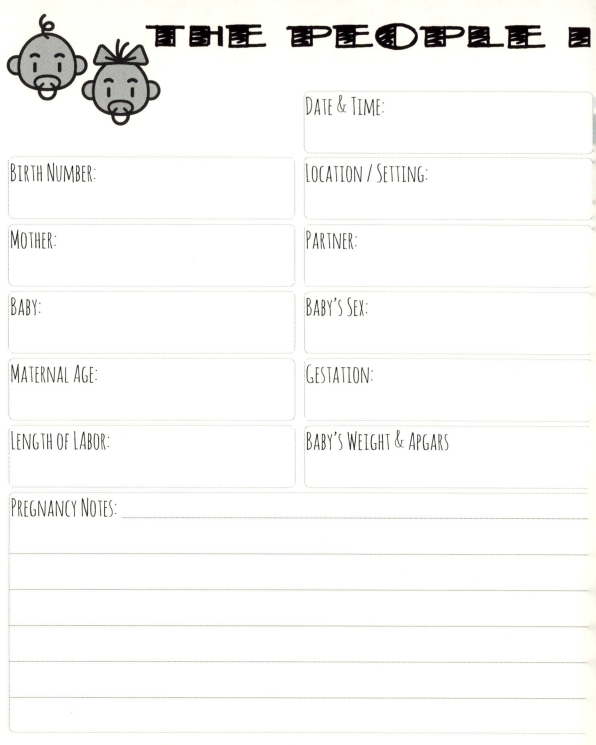

THE PEOPLE

Date & Time:

Birth Number:

Location / Setting:

Mother:

Partner:

Baby:

Baby's Sex:

Maternal Age:

Gestation:

Length of Labor:

Baby's Weight & Apgars

Pregnancy Notes:

HAVE HELPED OUT

COMMENTS:

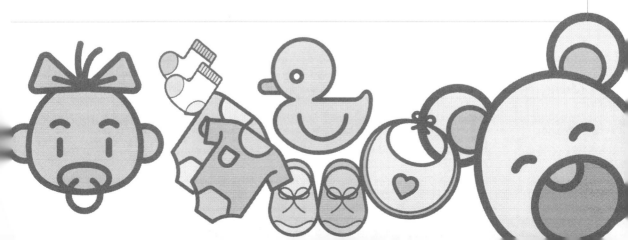

THE PEOPLE

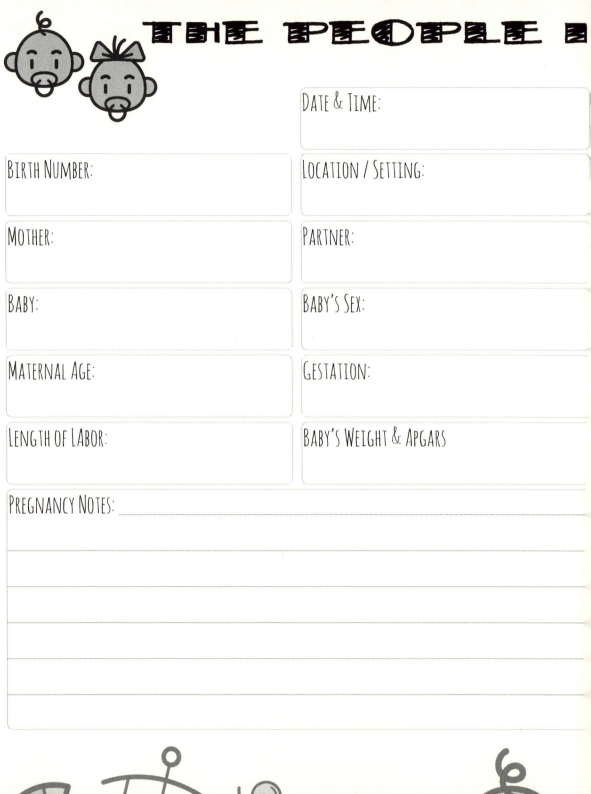

Date & Time:

Birth Number:

Location / Setting:

Mother:

Partner:

Baby:

Baby's Sex:

Maternal Age:

Gestation:

Length of Labor:

Baby's Weight & Apgars

Pregnancy Notes:

HAVE HELPED OUT

COMMENTS:

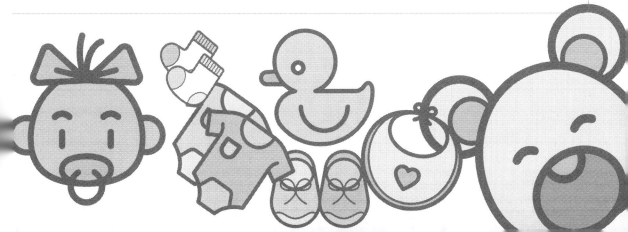

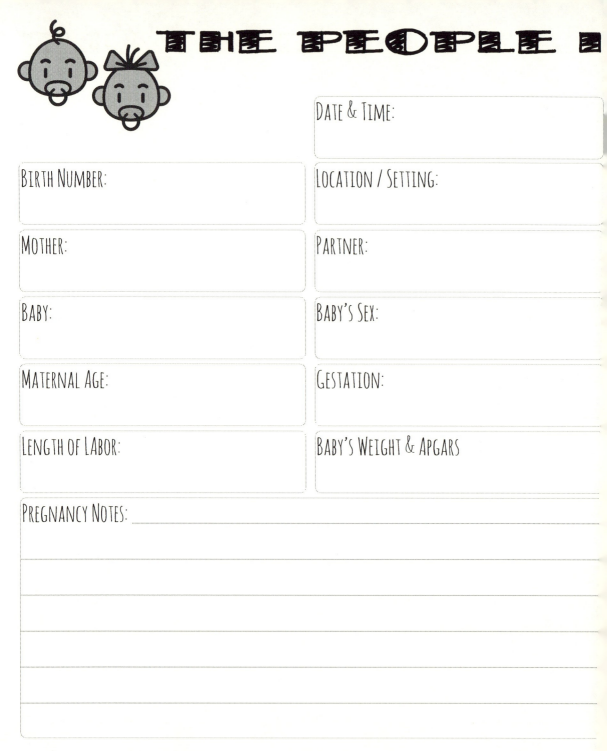

THE PEOPLE

Date & Time:

Birth Number:

Location / Setting:

Mother:

Partner:

Baby:

Baby's Sex:

Maternal Age:

Gestation:

Length of Labor:

Baby's Weight & Apgars

Pregnancy Notes:

HAVE HELPED OUT

COMMENTS:

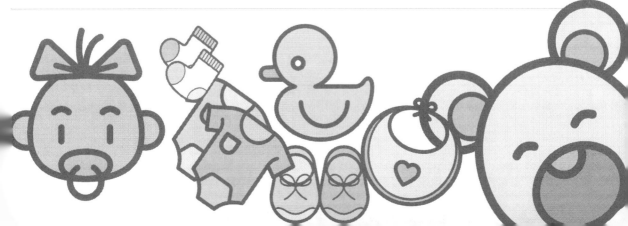

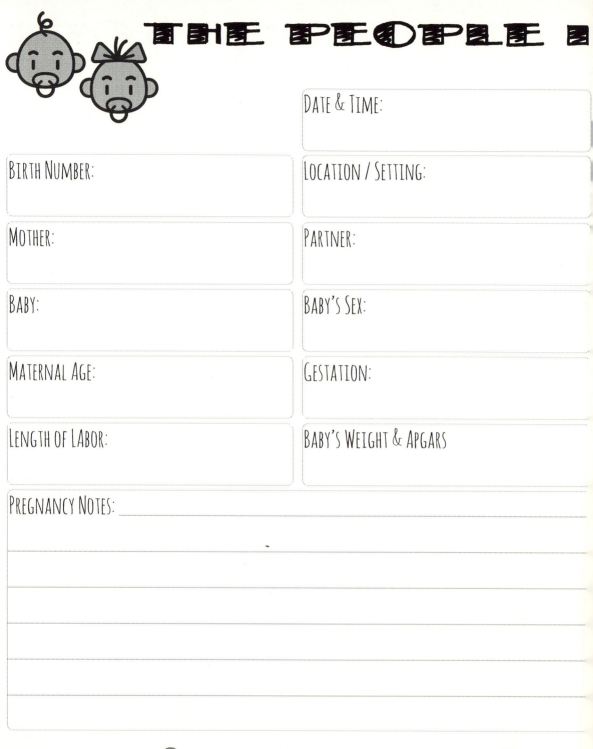

THE PEOPLE

Date & Time:

Birth Number:

Location / Setting:

Mother:

Partner:

Baby:

Baby's Sex:

Maternal Age:

Gestation:

Length of Labor:

Baby's Weight & Apgars

Pregnancy Notes:

HAVE HELPED OUT

COMMENTS:

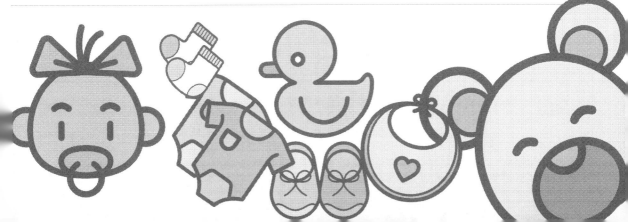

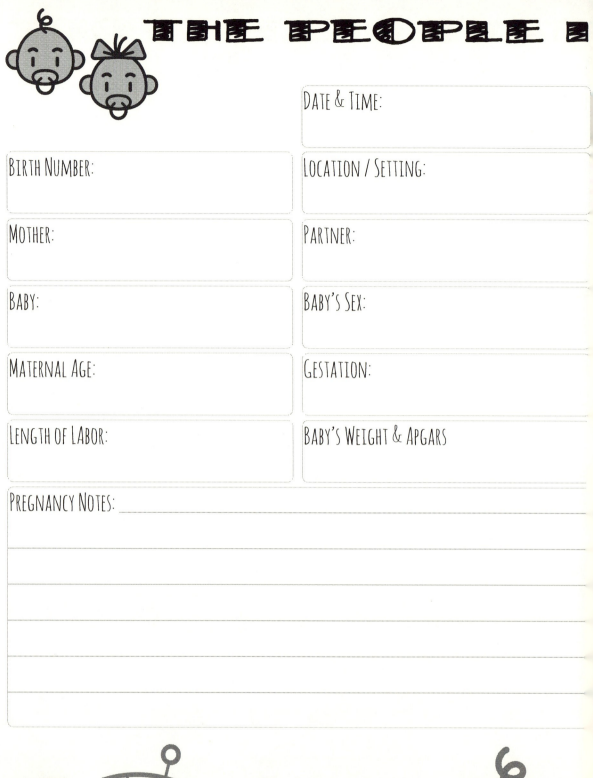

THE PEOPLE

Date & Time:

Birth Number:

Location / Setting:

Mother:

Partner:

Baby:

Baby's Sex:

Maternal Age:

Gestation:

Length of Labor:

Baby's Weight & Apgars

Pregnancy Notes:

HAVE HELPED OUT

COMMENTS:

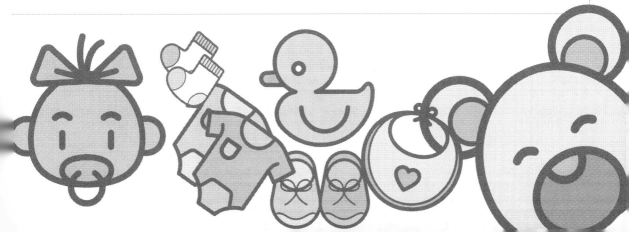

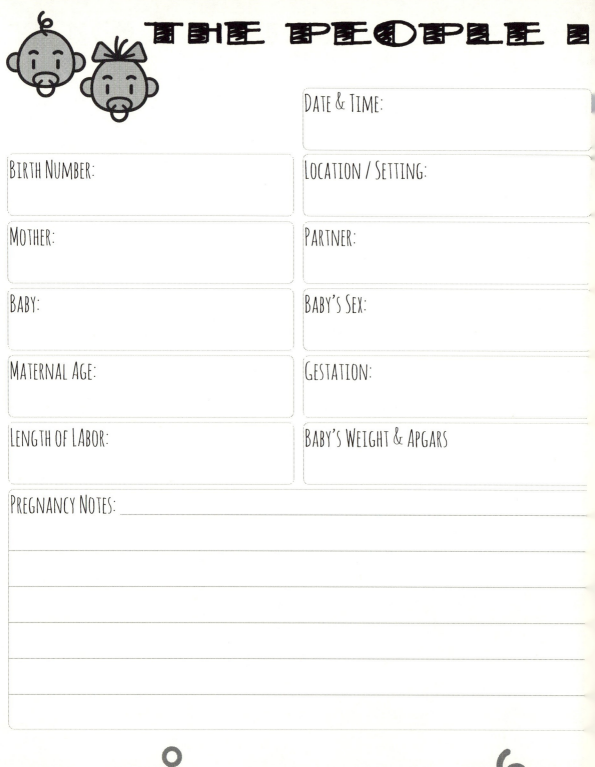

THE PEOPLE

Date & Time:

Birth Number:

Location / Setting:

Mother:

Partner:

Baby:

Baby's Sex:

Maternal Age:

Gestation:

Length of Labor:

Baby's Weight & Apgars

Pregnancy Notes:

HAVE HELPED OUT

COMMENTS:

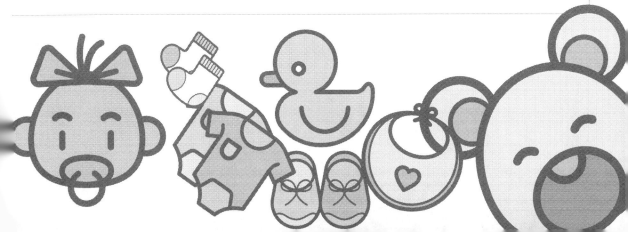

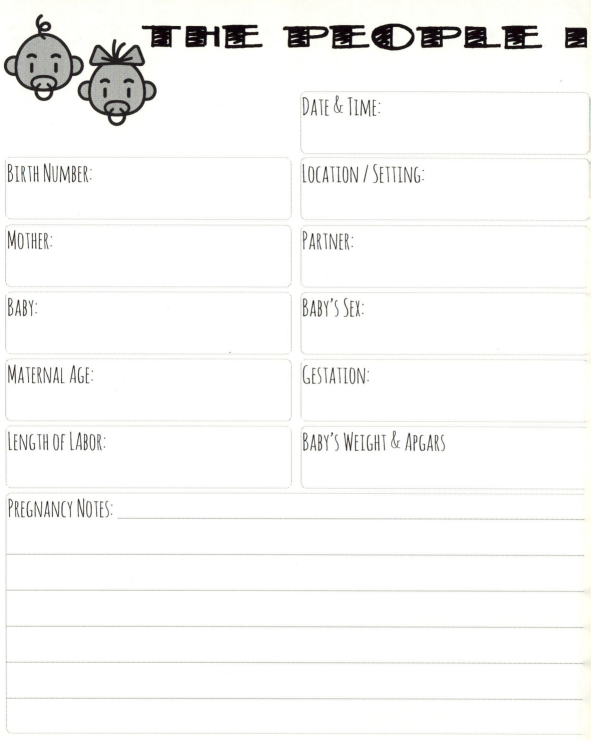

THE PEOPLE

Date & Time:

Birth Number:

Location / Setting:

Mother:

Partner:

Baby:

Baby's Sex:

Maternal Age:

Gestation:

Length of Labor:

Baby's Weight & Apgars

Pregnancy Notes:

HAVE HELPED OUT

COMMENTS:

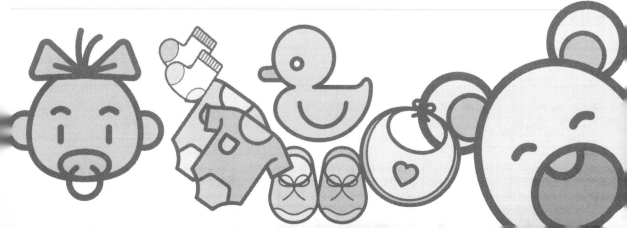

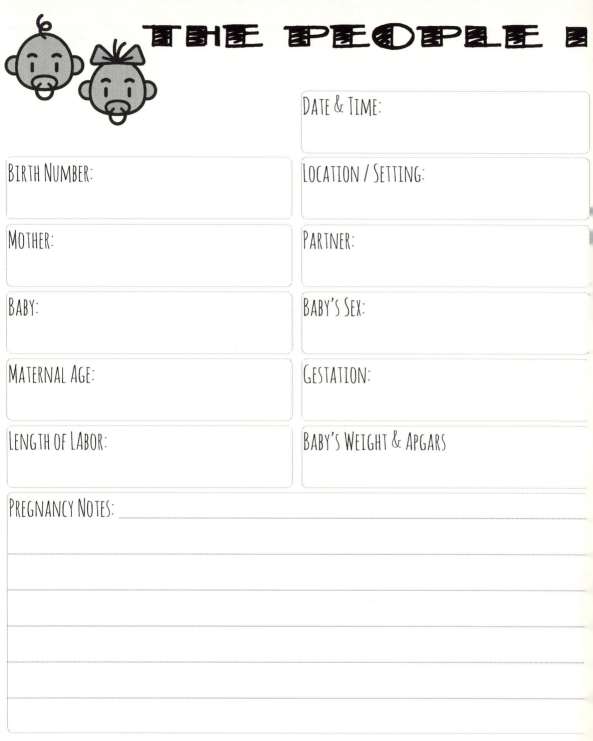

THE PEOPLE

Date & Time:

Birth Number:

Location / Setting:

Mother:

Partner:

Baby:

Baby's Sex:

Maternal Age:

Gestation:

Length of Labor:

Baby's Weight & Apgars

Pregnancy Notes:

HAVE HELPED OUT

COMMENTS:

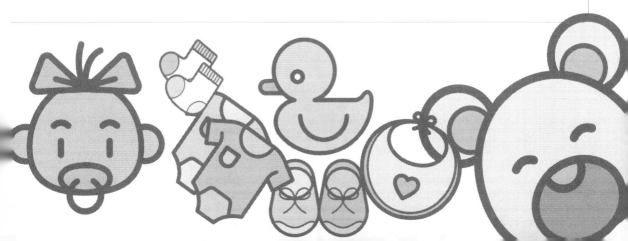

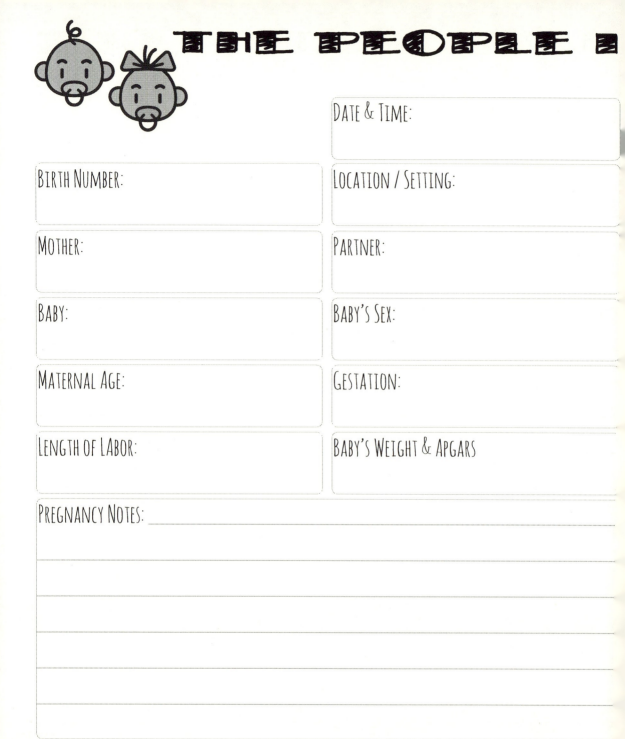

THE PEOPLE

Date & Time:

Birth Number:

Location / Setting:

Mother:

Partner:

Baby:

Baby's Sex:

Maternal Age:

Gestation:

Length of Labor:

Baby's Weight & Apgars

Pregnancy Notes:

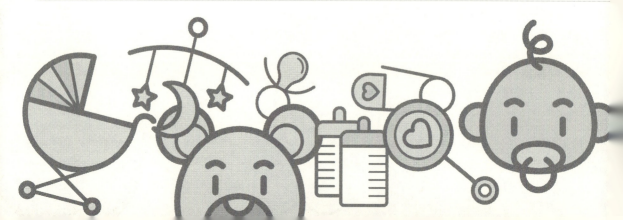

HAVE HELPED OUT

COMMENTS:

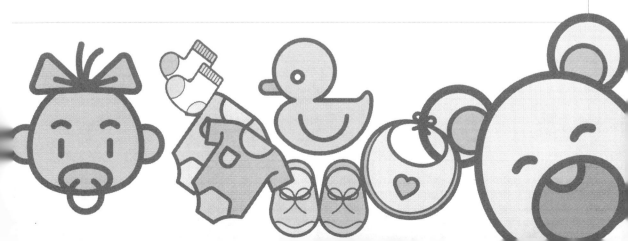

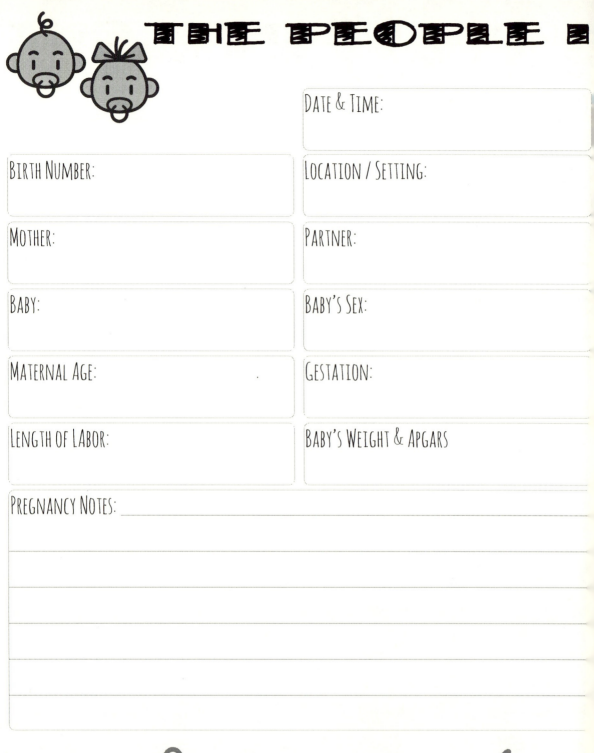

THE PEOPLE

Date & Time:

Birth Number:

Location / Setting:

Mother:

Partner:

Baby:

Baby's Sex:

Maternal Age:

Gestation:

Length of Labor:

Baby's Weight & Apgars

Pregnancy Notes:

HAVE HELPED OUT

COMMENTS:

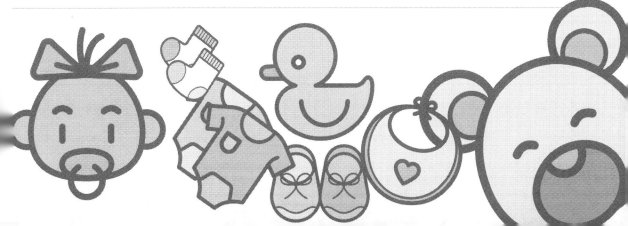

THE PEOPLE

Date & Time:

Birth Number:

Location / Setting:

Mother:

Partner:

Baby:

Baby's Sex:

Maternal Age:

Gestation:

Length of Labor:

Baby's Weight & Apgars

Pregnancy Notes:

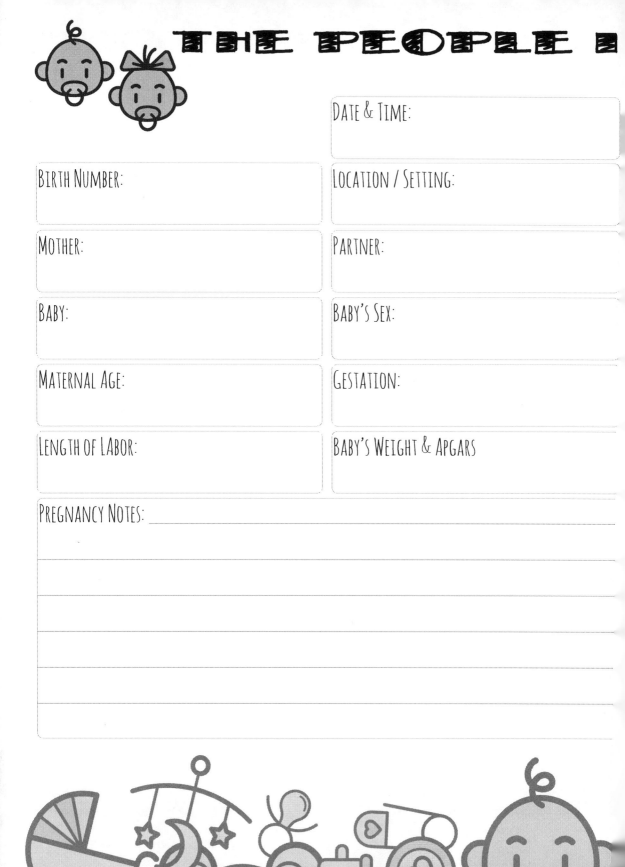

HAVE HELPED OUT

COMMENTS:

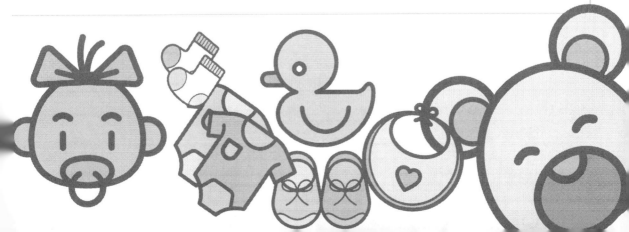

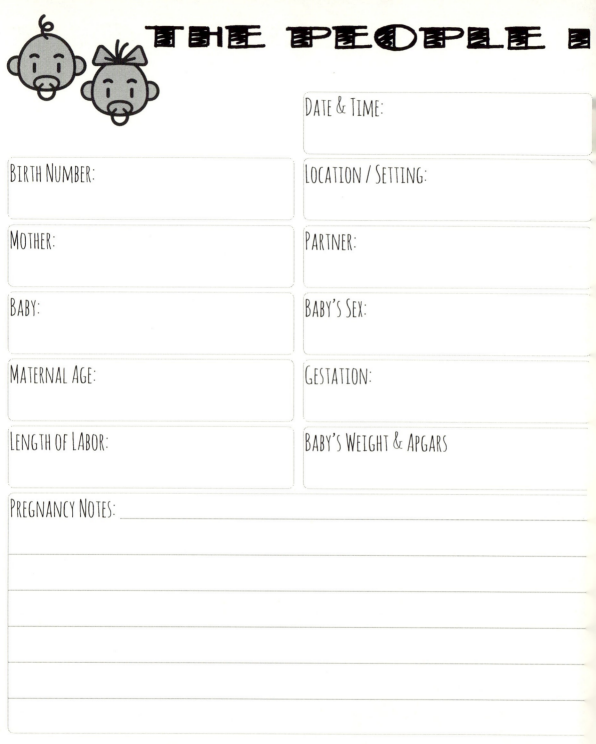

THE PEOPLE

Date & Time:

Birth Number:

Location / Setting:

Mother:

Partner:

Baby:

Baby's Sex:

Maternal Age:

Gestation:

Length of Labor:

Baby's Weight & Apgars

Pregnancy Notes:

HAVE HELPED OUT

COMMENTS:

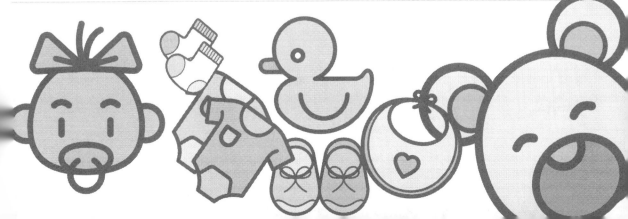

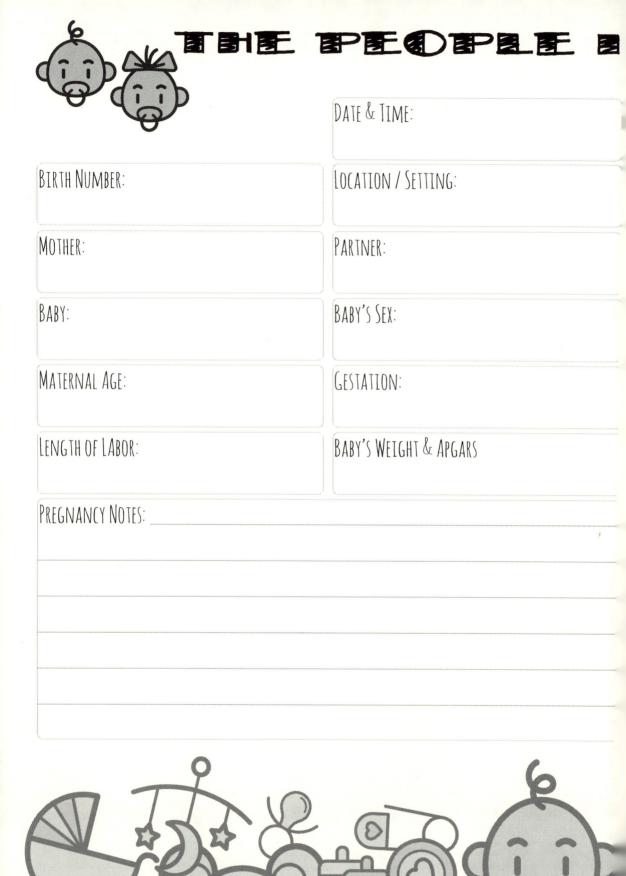

THE PEOPLE

Date & Time:

Birth Number:

Location / Setting:

Mother:

Partner:

Baby:

Baby's Sex:

Maternal Age:

Gestation:

Length of Labor:

Baby's Weight & Apgars

Pregnancy Notes:

HAVE HELPED OUT

COMMENTS:

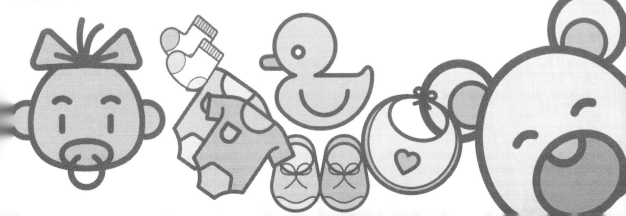

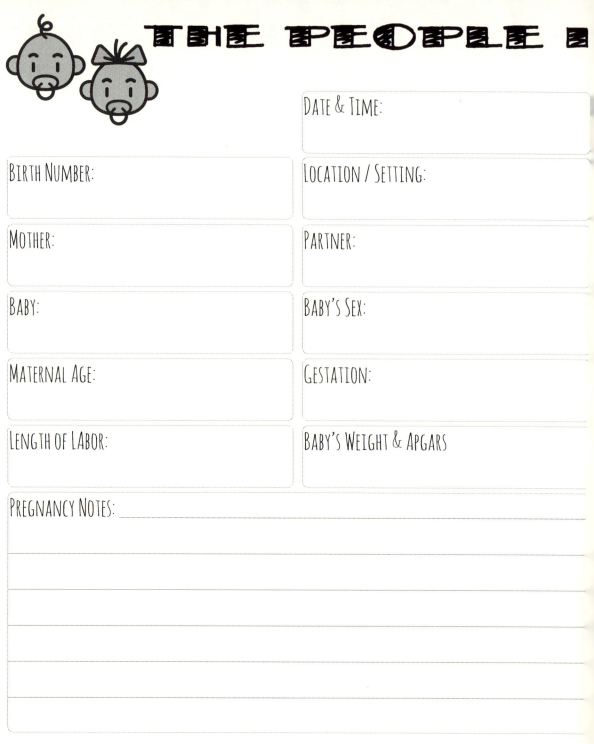

THE PEOPLE

DATE & TIME:

BIRTH NUMBER:

LOCATION / SETTING:

MOTHER:

PARTNER:

BABY:

BABY'S SEX:

MATERNAL AGE:

GESTATION:

LENGTH OF LABOR:

BABY'S WEIGHT & APGARS

PREGNANCY NOTES:

HAVE HELPED OUT

COMMENTS:

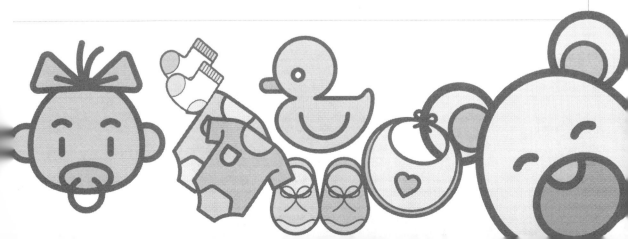

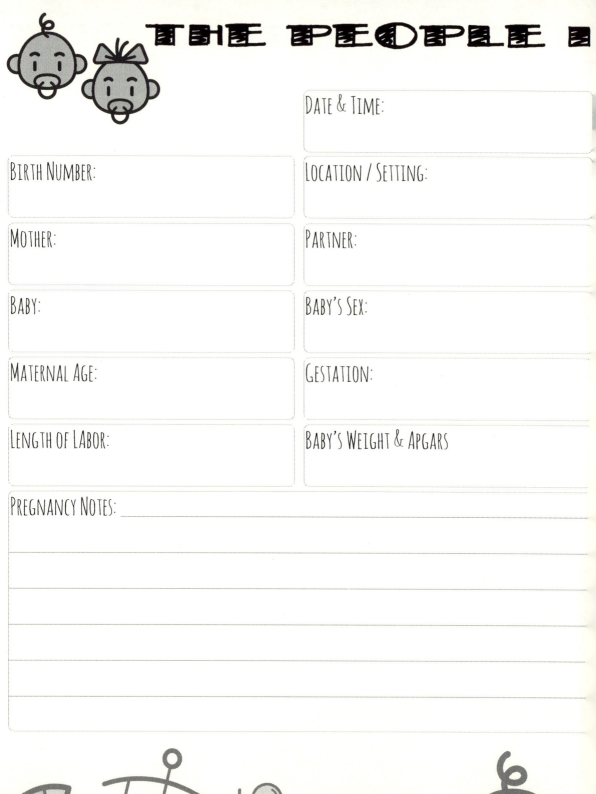

THE PEOPLE

Date & Time:

Birth Number:

Location / Setting:

Mother:

Partner:

Baby:

Baby's Sex:

Maternal Age:

Gestation:

Length of Labor:

Baby's Weight & Apgars

Pregnancy Notes:

HAVE HELPED OUT

COMMENTS:

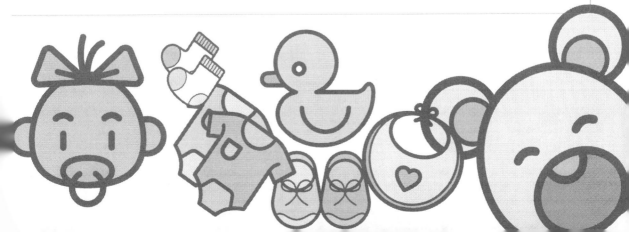

THE PEOPLE

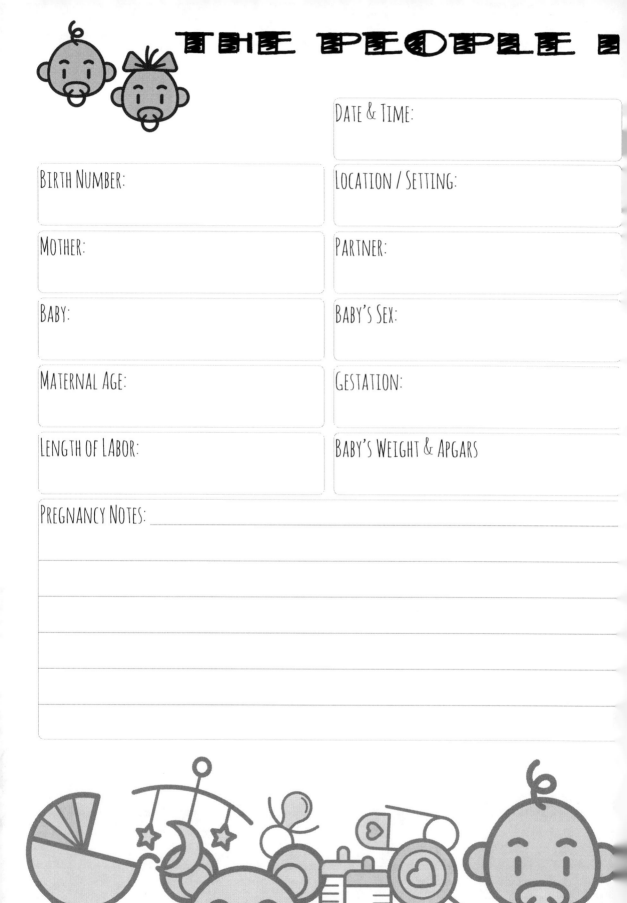

Birth Number:

Date & Time:

Location / Setting:

Mother:

Partner:

Baby:

Baby's Sex:

Maternal Age:

Gestation:

Length of Labor:

Baby's Weight & Apgars

Pregnancy Notes:

HAVE HELPED OUT

COMMENTS:

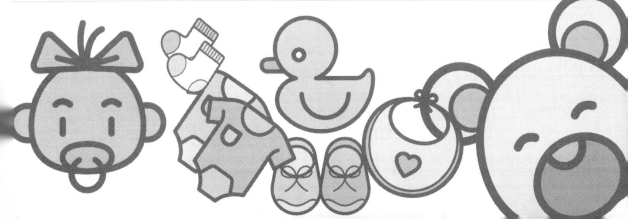

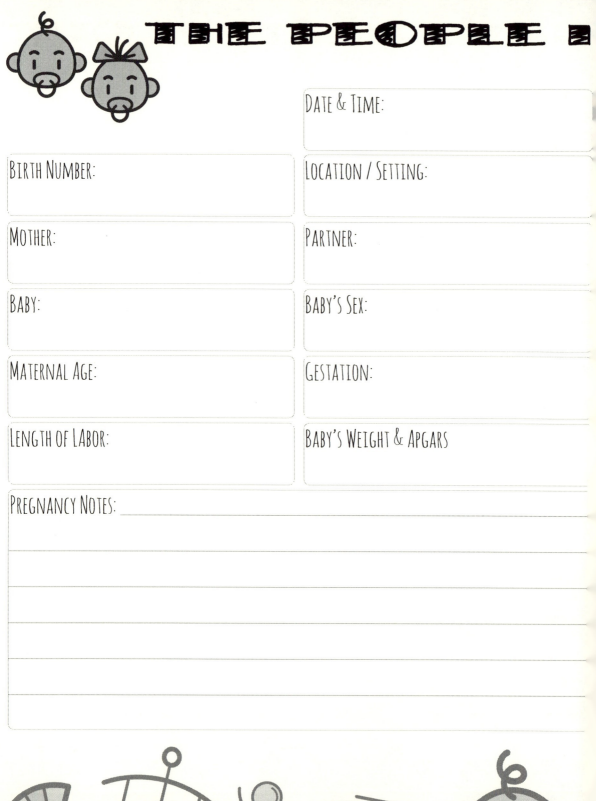

THE PEOPLE

Date & Time:

Birth Number:

Location / Setting:

Mother:

Partner:

Baby:

Baby's Sex:

Maternal Age:

Gestation:

Length of Labor:

Baby's Weight & Apgars

Pregnancy Notes:

HAVE HELPED OUT

COMMENTS:

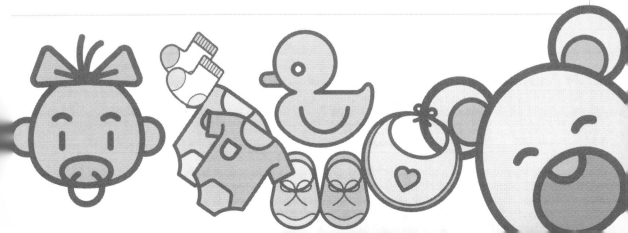

THE PEOPLE

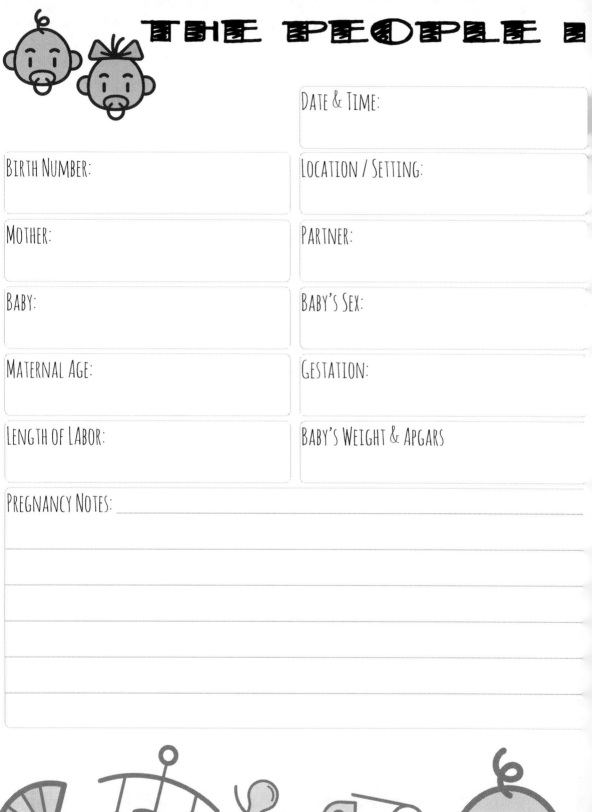

Date & Time:

Birth Number:

Location / Setting:

Mother:

Partner:

Baby:

Baby's Sex:

Maternal Age:

Gestation:

Length of Labor:

Baby's Weight & Apgars

Pregnancy Notes:

HAVE HELPED OUT

COMMENTS:

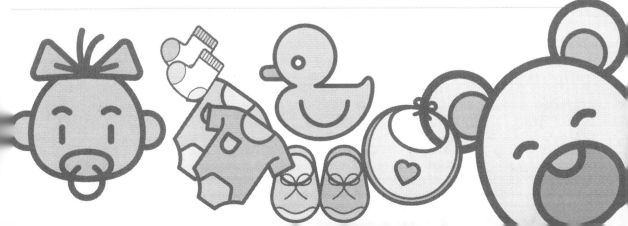

THE PEOPLE

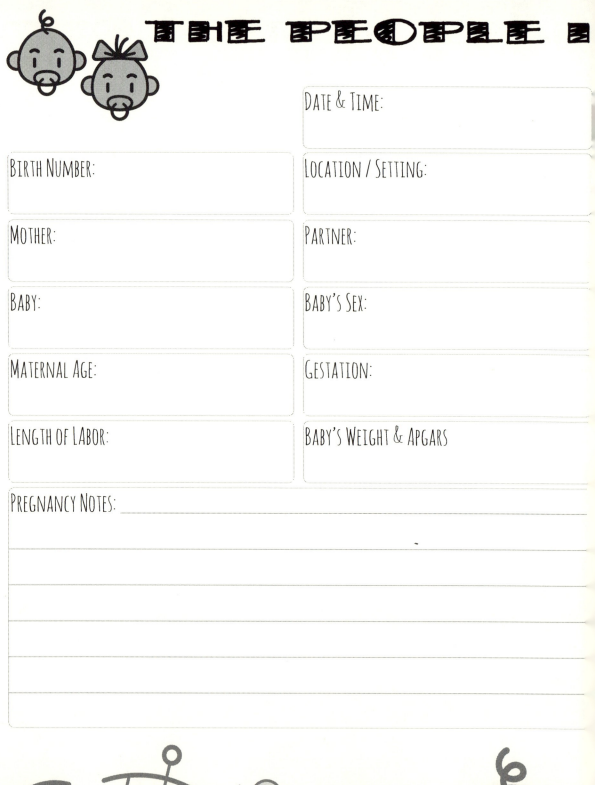

Date & Time:

Birth Number:

Location / Setting:

Mother:

Partner:

Baby:

Baby's Sex:

Maternal Age:

Gestation:

Length of Labor:

Baby's Weight & Apgars

Pregnancy Notes:

HAVE HELPED OUT

COMMENTS:

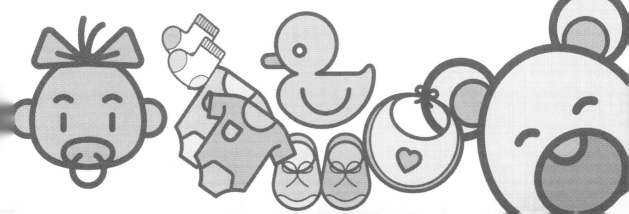

THE PEOPLE

Date & Time:

Birth Number:

Location / Setting:

Mother:

Partner:

Baby:

Baby's Sex:

Maternal Age:

Gestation:

Length of Labor:

Baby's Weight & Apgars

Pregnancy Notes:

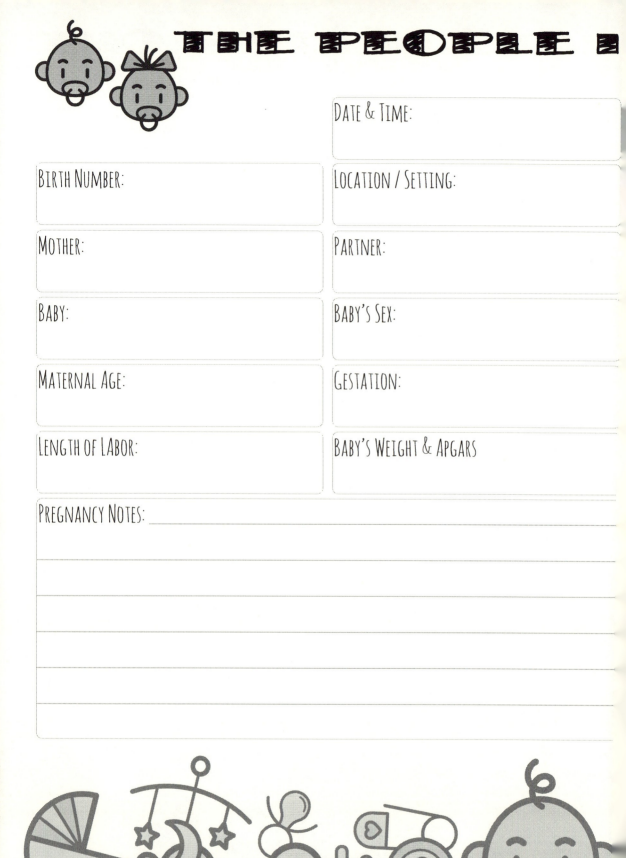

HAVE HELPED OUT

COMMENTS:

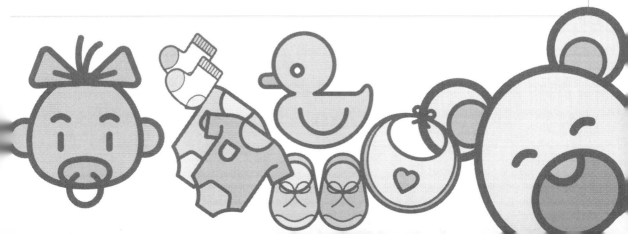

Made in the USA
Las Vegas, NV
29 January 2024

85019679R00072